Barbecue Cookbook

140 Of The Best
Barbecue Meat & Fish Recipes Book
With Recipe Journal

By: Samantha Michaels

TABLE OF CONTENTS

Publishers Notes 9

Dedication 10

Chapter 1- Beef Recipes 11

    Recipe 1 – Barbecue Bourbon Steak 11

    Recipe 2 – Tomato Herb Marinated Flank Steak 12

    Recipe 3 – Grilled Steak With A Whiskey And Dijon Sauce 14

    Recipe 4 – Grilled Thai Style Beef Kebabs 15

    Recipe 5 – Grilled Balsamic Steak 18

    Recipe 6 – Grilled Meatball Kebabs 20

    Recipe 7 – Easy Grilled Veal Chops 21

    Recipe 8 – Quick Grilled Beef Quesadillas 22

    Recipe 9 – Spicy Lime Marinated Round Eye Steaks 24

    Recipe 10 – Grilled Strip Steak With Garlic And Oregano 25

    Recipe 11 – Grilled Beef Tenderloin With A Herb, Garlic & Pepper Coating 26

    Recipe 12 – Beef In Hoisin And Ginger Sauce 27

    Recipe 13 – Ranch Burgers 29

    Recipe 14 – Three Herb Steak 30

    Recipe 15 – Peppered Rib Eye Steak 32

    Recipe 16 – Grilled Beef Tenderloin With Mediterranean Relish 34

Recipe 17 – Jerk Beef With Plantain Kebabs 36

Recipe 18 – Asian Barbecued Steak 37

Recipe 19 – Barbecued Chuck Roast 38

Recipe 20 – Barbecued Rib Eye Steak 40

Chapter 2- Chicken Recipes 42

Recipe 1 – Rotisserie Chicken 42

Recipe 2 – Shish Taouk Grilled Chicken 43

Recipe 3 – Grilled Butter Chicken 45

Recipe 4 – Blackened Chicken 47

Recipe 5 – Grilled Herb Chicken Burgers 48

Recipe 6 – Grilled Chicken Wing With Sweet Red Chili & Peach Glaze 49

Recipe 7 – Grilled Chicken Koftas 51

Recipe 8 – Thai Grilled Chicken With A Chili Dipping Sauce . 52

Recipe 9 – Catalan Chicken Quarters 54

Recipe 10 – Thai Chicken Satay 56

Recipe 11 – Barbecue Chicken Breasts 58

Recipe 12 – Spicy Plum Chicken Thighs 60

Recipe 13 – Maple Barbecued Chicken 62

Recipe 14 – Spatchcock Barbecue Chicken 63

Recipe 15 – Chicken Tikka Skewers 65

Recipe 16 – Sweet & Spicy Wings With Summer Coleslaw 67

Recipe 17 – Sticky Chicken Drumsticks 68

Recipe 18 – Jerk Chicken Kebabs And Mango Salsa 70

Recipe 19 – Chicken & Chorizo Kebabs With Chimichurri 72

Recipe 20 – Barbecued Chicken Burgers 73

Chapter 3- Pork Recipes 76

Recipe 1 – Pork Kebabs And Mushrooms 76

Recipe 2 – Barbecued Pork Steaks 77

Recipe 3 – Barbecued Pork Kebabs 79

Recipe 4 – Honey Mustard Pork Chops 80

Recipe 5 – Simple Grilled Pork Chops 82

Recipe 6 – Basic Barbecued Pork Spare Ribs 83

Recipe 7 – Southern Pulled Pork 85

Recipe 8 – Grilled Pork Tenderloin Satay 86

Recipe 9 – Easy Teriyaki Kebabs 88

Recipe 10 – Baby Back Barbecued Ribs 90

Recipe 11 – Maple Garlic Pork Tenderloin 91

Recipe 12 – Maple Glazed Ribs 93

Recipe 13 –Smoked Pork Spare Ribs 94

Recipe 14 – Bourbon Pork Ribs 97

Recipe 15 - Margarita Glazed Pork Chops 98

Chapter 4- Lamb Recipes 100

Recipe 1 – Lamb Chops With Curry, Apple And Raisin Sauce 100

Recipe 2 – Grilled Lamb With Brown Sugar Glaze 102

Recipe 3 – Mediterranean Lamb Burgers 103

Recipe 4 – Grilled Lamb Chops 105

Recipe 5 – Lamb Kofta Kebabs 107

Recipe 6 – Barbecued Asian Butterflied Leg Of Lamb 109

Recipe 7 – Summer Lamb Kebabs 111

Recipe 8 – Herb Marinated Lamb Chops 113

Recipe 9 – Grilled Indian Style Lamb Chops 114

Recipe 10 – Moroccan Leg of Lamb 116

Recipe 11 – South African Lamb And Apricot Sosaties (Kebabs) 117

Recipe 12 – Greek Lamb Chops 119

Recipe 13 – Grilled Rack Of Lamb 120

Recipe 14 – Greek Burgers 122

Recipe 15 – Teriyaki Lamb Kebabs 124

Chapter 5- Fish Recipes 127

Recipe 1 – Fresh Citrus Salmon 127

Recipe 2 – Marinated Barbecued Swordfish 129

Recipe 3 – Grilled Sea Bass With Garlic Sauce 130

Recipe 4 – Barbecued Salmon With Soy & Brown Sugar Marinade 132

Recipe 5 – Grilled Onion Butter Cod 133

Recipe 6 – Grilled Trout With Parsley 135

Recipe 7 – Barbecued Teriyaki Tuna Steaks 136

Recipe 8 – Lime & Basil Tilapia 138

Recipe 9 – Barbecued Tuna With Honey Glaze 139

Recipe 10 – Blackened Fish 141

Recipe 11 – Citrus Marjoram Marinated Halibut Steak..........142

Recipe 12 – Grilled Red Snapper 144

Recipe 13 – Ginger Swordfish 145

Recipe 14 – Grilled Asian Style Catfish 147

Recipe 15 – Barbecued Sea Bass 148

Recipe 16 – Grilled Trout In Corn Husks 150

Recipe 17 – Grilled Jamaican Jerk Catfish 151

Recipe 18 – Grilled Tandoori Cod 152

Recipe 19 – Grilled Mustard & Miso Sea Bass 154

Recipe 20 – Sea Bass Kebabs 156

Recipe 21 – Grilled Thai Red Snapper Packets 157

Recipe 22 – Moroccan Grilled Fish Kebabs 159

Recipe 23 – Grilled Fish Cakes 160

Recipe 24 – Tarragon Fish With Vegetables 162

Recipe 25 – Italian Style Trout 163

Recipe 26 – Perch With Sage 165

Recipe 27 – Sweet & Sour Halibut 166

Recipe 28 – Halibut & Red Pepper Kebabs 168

Recipe 29 – Fish Roll Ups 169

Recipe 30 – Grilled Snapper In A Banana Leaf 171

Recipe 31 – South Western Mahi Mahi 173

Recipe 32 – Grilled Shark 175

Recipe 33 – Grilled Catfish 176

Recipe 34 – Spicy Tuna Steaks 177

Recipe 35 – Asian Jerk Red Snapper 179

Recipe 36 – Grilled Fresh Sardines 180

Recipe 37 – Grilled Squid With Ginger, Celery & Apple Salad 182

Recipe 38 – Monkfish & Prawn Kebabs With Tomato Salsa 184

Recipe 39 – Skewered Swordfish With Charred Courgettes 187

Recipe 40 – Rosemary Salmon Burgers 189

Recipe 41 – Fast Fish Kebabs 191

Recipe 42 – Barbecued Halibut Steaks 192

Chapter 6- Shellfish Recipes 194

Recipe 1 – Grilled King Crab Legs 194

Recipe 2 – Spicy Shrimp Skewers 195

Recipe 3 – Grilled Oysters 197

Recipe 4 – Thai Spiced Prawns 198

Recipe 5 – Garlic Grilled Shrimps 200

Recipe 6 – Bacon Wrapped Shrimps 201

Recipe 7 – Scallops With A Herb & Pecan Crust 202

Recipe 8 – Grilled Oysters With Fennel Butter 204

Recipe 9 – Grilled Crab 205

Recipe 10 – Sesame Scallops 207

Recipe 11 – Margarita Shrimps 208

Recipe 12 – Baja Style Grilled Rock Lobster Tails 210

Recipe 13 – Grilled Prawns With Spicy Peanut Lime Vinaigrette 212

Recipe 14 – Scallops & Cherry Tomato Kebabs 214

Recipe 15 – Grilled Lobster with Lime Bay Butter 216

Recipe 16 – Grilled Prawns & Garlic Chili Sauce 217

Recipe 17 – Grilled New England Seafood 219

Recipe 18 – Honey Grilled Shrimps 221

Recipe 19 – Scallops Wrapped In Prosciutto 222

Recipe 20 – Maple Orange Shrimp & Scallop Kebabs 224

Recipe 21 – Ginger Shrimp with Charred Tomato Relish 225

Recipe 22 – Shrimp & Broccoli Packets 228

Recipe 23 – Tangy Shrimp & Scallops 229

Recipe 24 – Barbecued Oysters Served With Hogwash 231

Recipe 25 – Scallops, Orange & Cucumber Kebabs 232

Recipe 26 – Prawns With Pistou 233

Recipe 27 – Black & White Pepper Shrimps 235

Recipe 28 – Grilled Calamari 237

Recipe Journal 239

About The Author 260

PUBLISHERS NOTES

Disclaimer

This publication is intended to provide helpful and informative material. It is not intended to diagnose, treat, cure, or prevent any health problem or condition, nor is intended to replace the advice of a physician. No action should be taken solely on the contents of this book. Always consult your physician or qualified health-care professional on any matters regarding your health and before adopting any suggestions in this book or drawing inferences from it.

The author and publisher specifically disclaim all responsibility for any liability, loss or risk, personal or otherwise, which is incurred as a consequence, directly or indirectly, from the use or application of any contents of this book.

Any and all product names referenced within this book are the trademarks of their respective owners. None of these owners have sponsored, authorized, endorsed, or approved this book.

Always read all information provided by the manufacturers' product labels before using their products. The author and publisher are not responsible for claims made by manufacturers.

Paperback Edition

Manufactured in the United States of America

DEDICATION

This book is dedicated to people who enjoy food especially those who love to barbecue.

Chapter 1 - Beef Recipes

Recipe 1 – Barbecue Bourbon Steak

Although the flavor may be quite sweet, when teamed with a fresh crispy green salad you will find that this type of barbecued steak tastes wonderful.

Ingredients

4 x 200g Rump, Fillet or Sirloin Steaks

240ml Bourbon Whiskey

200g Dark Brown Sugar

Instructions

1. You need to lightly score the surface of each steak with the tip of a sharp knife on one side (diagonally). Then place into a shallow dish with the side you have scored facing upwards. Now you must pour the bourbon over the steaks and then over the top sprinkle on the dark brown sugar before then rubbing it in.

2. Once you have done the above you must now cover the steak up and place in the refrigerator and leave for 1 to 3 hours for the marinate to infuse into the meat. Around 15 minutes before you take the steaks out of the refrigerator you should get your barbecue going. Once the barbecue is hot enough and you have placed the grill about 6 inches above the heat you can place the steaks on to the grill sugar side down. Allow them to cook for around 4 to 5 minutes or until the sugar has caramelized.

3. Whilst the steak is going you should baste the side of the steak that is facing towards you with the remaining marinade before then turning it over. Just as with the previous side you should cook it again for around 4 to 5 minutes or cook until it is done to how you or your guests like it. Once the steak is ready serve immediately with a fresh green salad.

Recipe 2 – Tomato Herb Marinated Flank Steak

A very simple recipe that helps to make something that tastes truly amazing. If you can it is a good idea to allow the meat to remain in the marinade for at least 12 hours as this will help to make it much tender when it is cooked.

Ingredients

1 Medium Tomato

1 Shallot

60 ml Red Wine Vinegar

2 Tablespoons Fresh Chopped Marjoram

1 Tablespoon Fresh Chopped Rosemary

1 Teaspoon Salt

½ Teaspoon Freshly Ground Pepper

680 Grams Of Flank Steak

Samantha Michaels

Instructions

1. In a blender put the tomato, shallot (which have both been chopped), the marjoram, rosemary, salt and pepper. Blend until they form a smooth paste and set aside covered in the refrigerator. If there is any of the puree remaining in the blender scrape it out into a sealable plastic bag into which you then put the steak. Make sure that you spend time moving the steak around in the bag so that it is all coated in the puree. Once all the steak has been coated you now place it in the bag into the refrigerator and leave it to marinate for between 4 and 24 hours. The longer you leave the meat marinate in the puree the more flavor it will take on.

2. Once the allotted time has passed you should now get the barbecue heated up and set the grill above the heat at a height that it cooks the meat on a medium heat. Also make sure that you oil the rack first. Once the barbecue is heated up enough you should grill the steaks for between 4 to 5 minutes per side if you want yours medium rare or 6 to 7 minutes if you want yours to be medium. You should only turn the steaks one making sure that you brash the side that is already cooked with some of the sauce you reserved earlier.

3. As soon as the second side of the steak has been cooked you should turn it over again and brush it with more of the puree and then remove from the heat and place on a clean plate. Now allow it to rest for 5 minutes before then thinly cutting the steak crosswise. Before serving you should spoon on the rest of the puree.

Recipe 3 – Grilled Steak With A Whiskey And Dijon Sauce

Although this particular recipe contains alcohol when you cook it off you will find a lot of the whiskey taste has been removed instead a much sweeter oaky flavor is produced.

Ingredients

120ml Reduced Sodium Beef or Chicken Broth

3 Tablespoons Whiskey

3 Tablespoons Dijon Mustard

2 Tablespoons Light Brown Sugar

1 Large Shallot (Finely Chopped)

1 Teaspoon Worcestershire Sauce

1 Teaspoon Freshly Chopped Thyme

450 Gram Skirt Steak (Which has been trimmed and cut into 4 pieces)

½ Teaspoon Freshly Ground Pepper

¼ Teaspoon Salt

Instructions

1. Preheat your barbecue to a medium high heat. Whilst the barbecue is heating up you can prepare the sauce. To do this you

need to combine in a saucepan the whiskey, mustard, brown sugar, shallot, thyme and Worcestershire sauce. Bring all these ingredients to the boil then reduce the heat so that a lively simmer is maintained.

It is important that you stir this sauce frequently to prevent it sticking to the sides of the saucepan and burning. Keep it simmering for around 6 to 10 minutes until it has been reduced down by about half. Then remove from the heat.

2. Now you need to cook the steaks on the barbecue. But before you do sprinkle both sides with the salt and pepper. If you want yours to be medium you should cook each steak for between 1.5 and 3 minutes on each side. However you should cook them for less time if you want yours to be medium rare. Once they have been cooked for the recommended about of time remove them from the grill and let them rest for 5 minutes before serving with the sauce.

Recipe 4 – Grilled Thai Style Beef Kebabs

The use of Middle Eastern seasoning in these kebabs makes them taste absolutely wonderful as well as helping them to become much more tender when cooked.

Ingredients

450 gram Beef Sirloin (cut into 1 inch pieces)

1 Bell Pepper (cut into 1 inch pieces)

1 Small Onion (cut into 1 inch pieces)

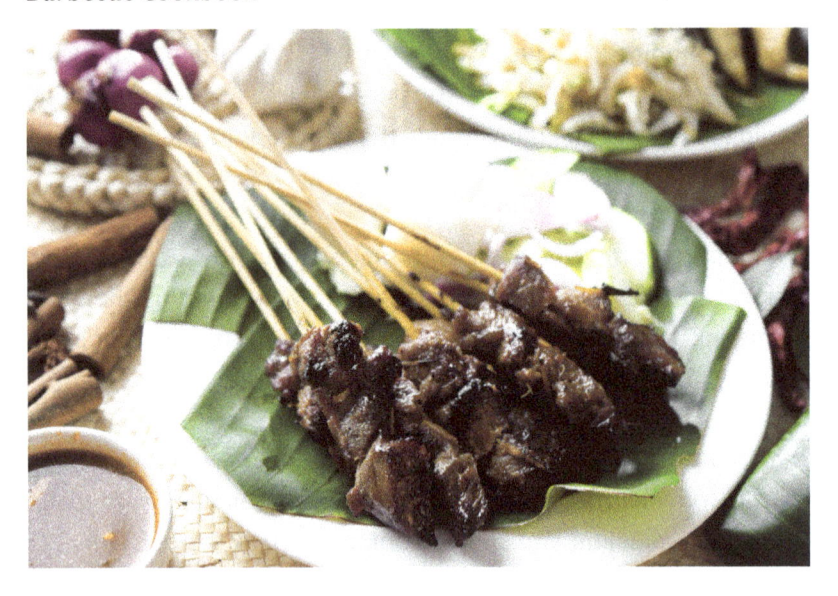

Marinade Ingredients

120ml Vegetable or Olive Oil

1 Tablespoon Rice Wine Vinegar

1 Tablespoon Roasted Sesame Seeds

2-3 Teaspoons Curry Powder

2 Teaspoons Soy Sauce

2 Teaspoons Sesame Oil

2 Gloves Minced Garlic

2 Teaspoons Dry Mustard

1 Teaspoon Hot Sauce

1 Teaspoon Cumin Powder

1 Teaspoon Sugar

½ Teaspoon Dried Ginger

½ Teaspoon Salt

½ Teaspoon Paprika

¼ Teaspoon Black Pepper

Instructions

1. Place the meat into a large sealable plastic bag and put to one side whilst you make the marinade. Best to place it in the refrigerator.

2. To make the marinade you combine all the ingredients above together in a bowl or jug. Once combined remove the meat from the refrigerator and pour the marinade directly into the bag and move the meat around to ensure that it is coated well. Replace the bag back in the refrigerator and leave it therefore for between 3 and 6 hours to allow the meat to become infused with the marinade.

3. When the allotted time has passed now remove the meat from the bag discarding it and the marinade. On to skewers you now place meat, onions and bell pepper alternately. If you are using wooden skewers then soak them in water for around 30 minutes, as this will prevent them from burning when placed on the barbecue.

4. To cook the kebabs place them on a grill over a medium to high heat and cook for 10 to 12 minutes, remembering to turn them occasionally. Once they are cooked remove from heat and serve.

RECIPE 5 – GRILLED BALSAMIC STEAK

If you are at all conscious about the number of carbs you are consuming then you will find this recipe ideal.

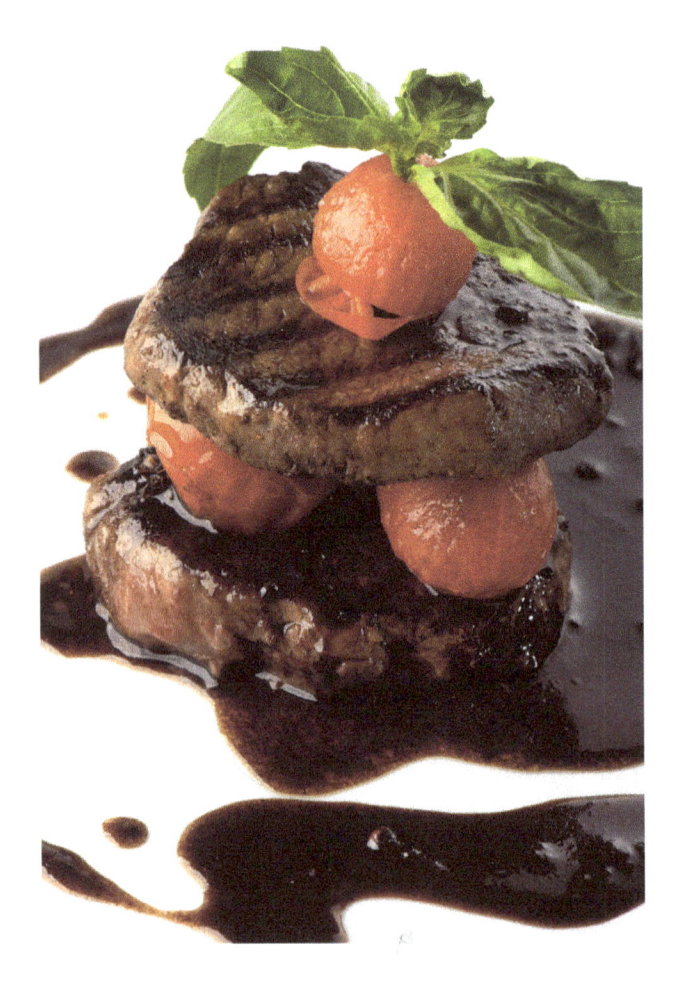

Ingredients

900gram Sirloin Steak (Should be about an inch thick)

240ml Water

120ml Soy Sauce

Samantha Michaels

1 Small Onion (minced)

2 Tablespoons Worcestershire Sauce

2 Tablespoons Balsamic Vinegar

1 Tablespoon Dijon Mustard

2 Gloves Garlic (minced)

¼ Teaspoon Hot Sauce

Instructions

1. Please the steak either into a glass dish or a bag that is sealable. Now combine the rest of the ingredients above in a bowl or a jug and whisk thoroughly.

2. Once you have combined all the ingredients above together you then pour of the steak and leave to marinate for between 1 and 12 hours. When you are ready to cook the steak you should get your barbecue heated up and cook it over a medium to high heat.

3. When the barbecue is at the right temperature you should remove the steak from the marinade and place it on the grill cooking it on each side for between 5 and 7 minutes if you like it medium. Any leftover marinade should be discarded and once the steak is cooked to the way you or your guests like it you can now remove it from the heat and serve.

Barbecue Cookbook

RECIPE 6 – GRILLED MEATBALL KEBABS

These meatball kebabs not only taste great when served on their own but also when you choose to put them into a sandwich.

Ingredients

450gram Ground Beef

1 Large Onion (cut into 1 inch pieces)

1 Large Red Or Yellow Bell Pepper (cut into 1 inch pieces)

115gram Dried Bread Crumbs

60ml Milk

75gram Parmesan Cheese (grated)

2 Gloves Garlic (Minced)

2 Tablespoons Dried Parsley

1 Tablespoon Dried Basil

½ Teaspoon Salt

½ Teaspoon Black Pepper

2 Eggs

Instructions

1. In a small bowl mix the bread crumbs and mil and let stand for 5 minutes. After five minutes squeeze the bread crumbs to help remove any excess milk and then combine this with the beef,

cheese, herbs, garlic, salt, pepper and eggs and blend them together well.

After combining all these ingredients together you shape the meat into around 16 to 18 meatballs. They should measure around ½ inch.

2. Once you have created the meatballs you place them onto skewers one at the time and in between each one place a piece of onion and pepper.

3. Now you need to place the kebabs on to your grill that is lightly oiled to prevent them from sticking and cook them on a medium heat for around 10 minutes. Remember to rotate them every 2 to 3 minutes to ensure that they are cooked evenly. Once they have been cooked properly you can remove them from the heat and serve.

RECIPE 7 – EASY GRILLED VEAL CHOPS

This is one of the simplest and easiest barbecue beef recipes you may want to try. It tastes absolutely delicious especially if you serve it with some freshly grilled vegetables.

Ingredients

6 Veal Chops (Should be about 1 ½ inches thick)

3 Tablespoons Extra Virgin Olive Oil

2 Teaspoons Freshly Chopped Thyme

½ Teaspoon Salt

½ Teaspoon Black Pepper

Instructions

1. Preheat heat the barbecue and cook the veal chops on a medium to high heat. Whilst the barbecue is heating up you can now prepare the chops.

2. The first thing you need to do is coat the veal chops in the olive oil before then sprinkling over them (both sides) the thyme, salt and pepper. Once you have done this you now place them on the barbecue grill and cook on each side for between 7 and 8 minutes. Once they have been cooked for the allotted time remove from heat and serve.

RECIPE 8 – QUICK GRILLED BEEF QUESADILLAS

The great thing about this particular recipe is that it doesn't take that long to prepare so makes the perfect food to have midweek or as a starter for when organizing a big barbecue that lots of friends and family are going to be attending.

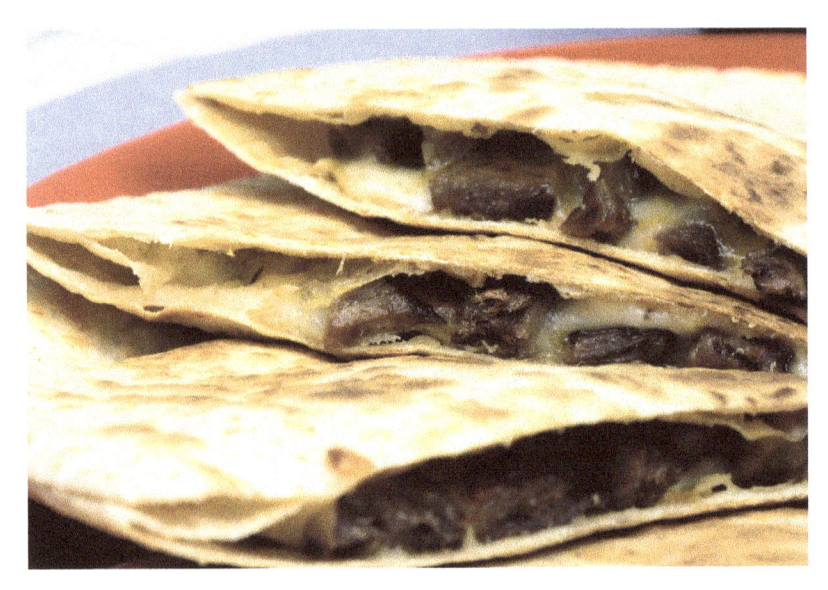

Samantha Michaels

Ingredients

229gram Sliced Roast Beef

1 Can Black Beans (drained and rinsed)

689gram Monterey Jack Cheese

8-10 Flour Tortillas

172gram Salsa

57gram Freshly Chopped Cilantro

3 Tablespoons Lime Juice

Instructions

1. Turn on the barbecue so it is heated up to the right temperature for you to then cook these quesadillas properly.

2. Whilst the barbecue is heating up in a bowl combine the salsa, cilantro and lime juice and then set to one side. However before you do set it aside mix a third of this mixture with the beans in a separate bowl.

3. Now you are ready to start making the quesadillas. Onto one of the tortillas place some of the sliced roast beef and cheese before then topping off with a spoonful of the beans and salsa mix. Fold the tortilla over and place on the barbecue grill and cook for between 4 and 5 minutes turning them over once. Remove them from the heat as they turn golden brown and serve with the other salsa mix you made earlier.

Recipe 9 – Spicy Lime Marinated Round Eye Steaks

Another barbecued beef recipe that doesn't require a lot of preparation, but will still produce wonderful tasting food. Best served with grilled potatoes or a fresh green salad.

Ingredients

2 x 226gram Round Eye Steaks (measuring 1 inch thick)

Juice from 1 Lime

1 Teaspoon Garlic Powder

1 Teaspoon Cumin Powder

1 Teaspoon Ground Coriander

1 Teaspoon Salt

1 Teaspoon Freshly Ground Pepper

Instructions

1. In a bowl combine together the lime juice, garlic powder, cumin, coriander, salt and pepper.

2. Next trim of any fat that is visible from the steaks and place them in a plastic bag that can be resealed. But before closing the bag up pour in the mix you made earlier ensuring that the steaks have been coated well and leave in the refrigerator for 30 minutes.

3. Whilst the steaks are marinating you can start heating up the grill ready for cooking. Once the 30 minutes has passed you can

remove the steaks from the bag and place them on the grill. Cook each side of the steak for 4 to 5 minutes before serving them.

Recipe 10 – Grilled Strip Steak With Garlic And Oregano

Another barbecued steak recipe that doesn't need a lot of preparation and so can be prepared and served to your guests very quickly.

Ingredients

4 Strip Steaks (1 Inch Thick)

3 Gloves Of Garlic Minced

1 ½ Tablespoons Olive Oil

1 Tablespoon Dried Crushed Oregano

¼ Teaspoon Salt

¼ Teaspoon Freshly Ground Pepper

Instructions

1. In a small bowl combine together the oil, garlic, oregano, salt and pepper then slather over the steak on both sides. Then place them in a dish that you cover and put in the refrigerator for 2 to 3 hours to allow the steak to become infused with the marinate.

Barbecue Cookbook

2. It is important that when cooking these steaks you do so on the highest heat possible on the barbecue. Place them on the barbecue grill and cook each site for between 6 to 8 minutes. Once both sides have been cooked remove from heat and serve.

Recipe 11 – Grilled Beef Tenderloin With A Herb, Garlic & Pepper Coating

You may want to consider trying out this recipe first before you decide to serve to your guests. This will then help to ensure that you cook the meat properly.

Ingredients

2.26Kg Whole Beef Tenderloin

6 Tablespoons Olive Oil

8 Large Garlic Cloves Minced

2 Tablespoons Freshly Minced Rosemary

1 Tablespoon Dried Thyme Leaves

2 Tablespoons Coarsely Ground Black Pepper

1 Tablespoon Salt

Instructions

1. You need to prepare the beef first. This means trimming off any excess fat with a sharp knife before folding over the thinnest part of the meat so that it is about the same thickness as the rest. Of

course if you want you could ask your butcher to do this for you. They will then tie it with butchers twine as well. It is also important that you snip the silver skin on the meat, as this will prevent it from bowing when it is cooking.

2. Once the meat is prepared now you need to mix the other ingredients together and then rub these all over the meat. Place the meat in the refrigerator whilst you prepare the barbecue to cook it on. If you are using a charcoal grill then build the fire on just one half of it. However if you are using a gas barbecue turn the burners up high for 10 minutes.

3. Before you place the meat on to the grill make sure that you coat it well with oil using a cloth that is soaked in oil between a pair of tongs. Once the grill has been coated with oil place the beef onto it and close the lid. After 5 minutes you now need to turn the meat over and repeat the same process.

4. After the meat has been seared (sealed) on both sides you now need to place it on to the side of the charcoal grill which is cooler or if using a gas barbecue turn off the heat directly underneath the meat. Cook for around 45 to 60 minutes or when a thermometer is inserted the internal temperature of the beef has reached 130 degrees Fahrenheit. Once it has cooked for the time stated now remove if from the heat and let it stand for 15 minutes (cover it over) before carving.

RECIPE 12 – BEEF IN HOISIN AND GINGER SAUCE

Looking for something with a little kick, then look no further than this particular recipe. You can either serve this with some rice or noodles or some grilled Pak Choi.

Barbecue Cookbook

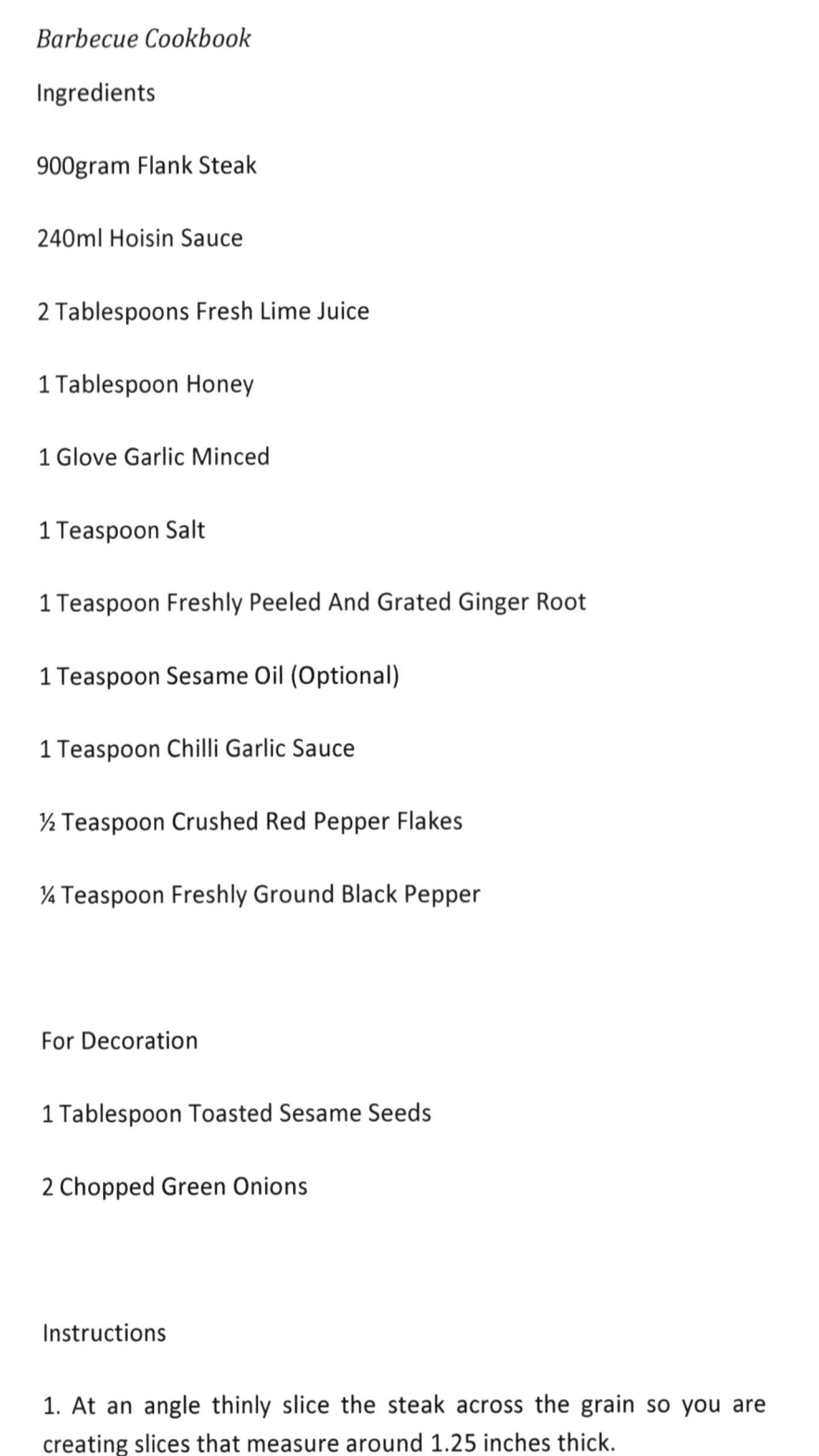

Ingredients

900gram Flank Steak

240ml Hoisin Sauce

2 Tablespoons Fresh Lime Juice

1 Tablespoon Honey

1 Glove Garlic Minced

1 Teaspoon Salt

1 Teaspoon Freshly Peeled And Grated Ginger Root

1 Teaspoon Sesame Oil (Optional)

1 Teaspoon Chilli Garlic Sauce

½ Teaspoon Crushed Red Pepper Flakes

¼ Teaspoon Freshly Ground Black Pepper

For Decoration

1 Tablespoon Toasted Sesame Seeds

2 Chopped Green Onions

Instructions

1. At an angle thinly slice the steak across the grain so you are creating slices that measure around 1.25 inches thick.

2. Next in a bowl whisk together the hoisin sauce, lime juice, honey, garlic, salt, sesame oil, chili garlic sauce, red pepper flakes and pepper. Then pour into a plastic resealable bag and into this also put the steak and move it around so it is well coated by the marinade. Then place in the refrigerator for between 2 to 12 hours to allow the meat to become infused with the marinade.

3. When you want to cook the steak you should preheat your barbecue to a medium to high heat and thread the slices of meat on to skewers. If you are using wooden skewers soak them in water for around 30 minutes, as this will prevent them from burning when you place them on the grill. Any leftover marinade should then be discarded.

4. Cook the meat on the barbecue for between 2 and 3 minutes on each side depending on how you like your beef to be cooked. 2 minutes for rare to medium and 3 minutes for well done. Once the steak has been cooked sprinkle them with the toasted sesame seeds and chopped green onions before serving.

RECIPE 13 – RANCH BURGERS

This is a very quick and easy way to make burgers that not only taste wonderful but also look wonderful as well. Because very little preparation is involved you may want to consider getting your kids to help you make them.

Ingredients

900gram Lean Ground Beef

1 Pack of Ranch Dressing Mix

Barbecue Cookbook

1 Egg (Lightly Beaten)

172gram Saltine Crackers (Crushed)

1 Onion (Chopped)

Instructions

1. In to a bowl place the ground beef, the dressing mix, the egg, crushed crackers and onion. Combine well together before then forming them into hamburger patties. You should be making the burgers as you allow the barbecue to heat up to a high temperature.

2. Once the burgers are ready and the barbecue has reached the desired you now place them on it. It is a good idea to coat the grill with some oil first to prevent the burgers stick to it. You should cook each side of the burger for 5 minutes and when done you serve them in a sesame topped bun.

RECIPE 14 – THREE HERB STEAK

A very simple and quick recipe to prepare but the herbs used help to bring out even more of the steaks flavor. Ideal for serving to those who don't like their food a little hot.

Ingredients

2 Beef Top Loin Steaks (1 ½ Inch Thick)

Samantha Michaels

2 Medium Red or Yellow Sweet Peppers (Seeds Removed And Cut Into ½ Inch Rings)

1 Tablespoon Olive Oil

Salt And Pepper To Season

Marinade

114gram Freshly Cut Parsley

60ml Olive Oil

57gram Freshly Cut Basil

1 Tablespoon Freshly Cut Oregano

1 to 2 Teaspoons Of Freshly Cracked Black Pepper

½ Teaspoon Salt

Instructions

1. In a bowl mix the olive oil, basil, parsley, oregano, cracked black pepper and salt to create the marinade.

2. Before rubbing the mixture made up over the steak (both sides) you need to trim off any fat. Once coated in the marinade you need to place them on a clean plate (covered) and put in the refrigerator for one hour.

3. Whilst the steak is in the refrigerator slice up the pepper before then coating with olive oil, salt and pepper. Put these to one side ready for when you start cooking.

Barbecue Cookbook

4. As soon as you remove the steak from the refrigerator start up the barbecue. This will allow time for the meat to come up to room temperature making it much easier to cook. If you want your steaks to be medium rare cook for between 15 and 19 minutes (turning once during this time). However if you want your steaks to be medium then cook for between 18 and 23 minutes. Put the peppers on to grill around 10 minutes before you take the meat off. You should turn them once during this time to sure that they are cooked well.

5. After the time for cooking the steaks has passed remove from heat place on a clean plate sprinkle with rest of herb mixture before covering and leaving to stand for 10 minutes. To serve you simple slice the steak across the grain and then top off with some of the pepper rings.

RECIPE 15 – PEPPERED RIB EYE STEAK

Applying the dry rub mixture to the meat before cooking helps to make it taste more succulent. Plus it also helps to reduce the amount of calories and fat you are consuming.

Ingredients

4 x 285-340gram Rib Eye Steaks (Cut 1 Inch Thick)

1 Tablespoon Olive Oil

1 Tablespoon Paprika

1 Tablespoon Garlic Powder

2 Teaspoons Crushed Dried Thyme

Samantha Michaels

2 Teaspoons Crushed Dried Oregano

1 ½ Teaspoons Lemon Pepper Seasoning

1 Teaspoon Salt

½ to 1 Teaspoon Freshly Ground Black Pepper

½ to 1 Teaspoon Cayenne Pepper

Instructions

1. Trim any excess fat from the steak then brush with the olive oil. Also snip the edges of the steak before coating to prevent them curling up when grilling on the barbecue.

2. In a bowl combine the other ingredients together before then sprinkling over the meat evenly before then rubbing it into the meat with your fingers. Place on a clean plate and cover the steaks once both sides have been coated in the dry mixture before then placing in a refrigerator for 1 hour.

3. To cook the steaks remove from refrigerator whilst the barbecue is heating up and when ready cook them directly over a medium heat and cook until they are done to the way you and your guests like to eat them. For steaks that are medium rare cook for between 11 and 15 minutes, turning them once. Whilst if you want yours cooked to medium then keep then on the grill for between 14 and 18 minutes. Again turning them over once during this time.

Recipe 16 – Grilled Beef Tenderloin With Mediterranean Relish

The Mediterranean Relish that you make to go with this particular barbecued beef dish really helps to create a more summery feel to the meal.

Ingredients

1.3to1.8Kg Center Cut Beef Tenderloin

2 Japanese Eggplants (Cut Lengthwise In Half)

2 Red Or Yellow Sweet Peppers (Seeded and Cut Lengthwise in Half)

1 Sweet Onion (Cut Into ½ Inch Slices)

2 Plum Tomatoes (Chopped)

2 Tablespoons Kalamata Olives (Pipped and Chopped)

2 Tablespoons Olive Oil

2 Teaspoons Crushed Dried Oregano

2 Teaspoons Cracked Black Pepper

1 ½ Teaspoons Freshly Shredded Lemon Peel

3 Cloves Garlic (Minced)

2 Tablespoons Freshly Snipped Basil

1 Tablespoon Balsamic Vinegar

¼ to ½ Teaspoon Salt

1/8 Teaspoon Ground Black Pepper

Instructions

1. In a small bowl combine together the cracked black pepper, lemon peel, oregano, and 2 of the minced garlic cloves. Once thoroughly combined together rub this all over the meat.

2. To cook the meat you need to place a drip tray in the bottom of the barbecue and around it place the hot charcoal. Once the temperature has reached the right level place the meat on the grill above the drip tray. As for the vegetables these should be placed around the meat directly over the coals, brushing them with olive oil first. Close the lid on the grill and allow it to remain closed for 10 to 12 minutes. By this time the vegetables should be tender and need to be removed from the grill.

3. Once the vegetables have been removed and placed on a clean plate and covered close the lid on the barbecue once more and allow the meat to continue cooking for between 25 and 30 minutes or until the internal temperature of the meat has reached 135 degrees Fahrenheit when a meat thermometer is inserted. If this temperature has been reached remove meat from barbecue place on a clean plate and cover leaving it to rest for 15 minutes before you slice it.

4. Now the vegetables have had sufficient time to cool down you can make the relish to go with the beef. Simply put all the vegetables into a bowl after coarsely chopping them and add to them the olives, basil, tomatoes, and garlic clove, vinegar, salt and ground black pepper.

Recipe 17 – Jerk Beef With Plantain Kebabs

You may think combining Plantain (a form of banana) with beef seems wrong, but the use of the Jamaican jerk seasoning helps to combat this.

Ingredients

340gram Boneless Sirloin Steak (Cut To 1 Inch Thick)

2 Tablespoons Red Wine Vinegar

1 Tablespoon Cooking Oil (Vegetable Is Best)

1 Tablespoon Jamaican Jerk Seasoning

2 Ripe Plantains (Peeled Then Cut Into 1 Inch Chunks)

1 Medium Sized Red Onion (Cut Into Wedges)

Instructions

1. Trim any excess fat from the meat before then cutting into 1 inch thick pieces then place to one side whilst you make the marinade for it.

2. Into a bowl place the vinegar, oil and jerk seasoning. Use a whisk to make sure that all the ingredients have been combined well together. Now divide the mixture into two separate amounts and use one half of the mixture to coat the steak. Then leave the steak to marinate in this mixture whilst you prepare the plantain and onion to make the skewers.

3. To make the kebabs you thread on to them meat, plantain and onion. Make sure you leave a gap of about ¼ inch between each item placed on the skewer. Then brush the onions and plantain with the other half of the marinade mixture.

4. In order to cook the kebabs you place them directly over the coals or turn the burners down to a medium heat and grill for between 12 and 15 minutes. It is important that you turn the kebabs occasionally to ensure that they are cooked evenly.

Recipe 18 – Asian Barbecued Steak

You may find the thought of combining fish sauce with beef a little off putting. However when combined with the other ingredients in this recipe it helps to make the meat much more flavorsome and tender.

Ingredients

907gram Flank Steak

60ml Chilli Sauce

60ml Fish Sauce

1 ½ Tablespoons Dark Sesame Oil

1 Tablespoon Freshly Grated Ginger Root

2 Gloves Garlic (Peeled And Crushed)

Instructions

1. In to a bowl pour the chilli sauce, fish sauce, sesame oil, grated ginger root and garlic and mix well together. Now set aside a few tablespoons of this mixture, as you will use it to baste the meat whilst it is on the barbecue.

2. Next you must score the meat and then place it in a shallow dish before then pouring over the remainder of the marinade you made earlier. Turn the meat over to ensure that it coated in the sauce completely. Then cover the meat and place in the refrigerator for no less than 3 hours.

3. To cook the steak you need to heat the barbecue up to a high temperature. Then just before placing the meat on to the barbecue brush the grill lightly with oil to prevent the meat from sticking to it. Now grill the meat for around 5 minutes on each side to have meat that is medium rare. Of course if you want your meat to be cooked to medium or well done levels then cook on each side for a little cooker. Whilst cooking brush over some more of the marinade you put to one side. When cooked let stand for a few minutes before then serving.

RECIPE 19 – BARBECUED CHUCK ROAST

Still hunkering after a roast dinner in the summer then this is a very quick and easy way of doing it. Plus doing it on the barbecue means much less mess for you to clear up in doors.

Ingredients

2.2 Kg Chuck Roast

240ml Barbecue Sauce

240ml Teriyaki Sauce

350ml Beer (Canned Or Bottled)

3 Teaspoons Minced Garlic

3 Teaspoons Freshly Thinly Sliced Ginger Root

1 Onion (Finely Chopped)

3 Teaspoons Coarsely Ground Black Pepper

2 Teaspoons Salt

Instructions

1. Into a large bowl mix together the barbecue sauce with the teriyaki sauce, beer, garlic, ginger, onion, coarsely ground black pepper and salt. Then place the roast into the marinade just made, cover and put into the refrigerator for 6 hours. It is important that turn the meat often whilst in the refrigerator to ensure that all of it is well coated.

2. You need to preheat your barbecue to allow you to cook the meat using the indirect heat method. Once the barbecue has had sufficient time to heat up now remove the meat from the marinade before then place on the barbecue grill on thread onto a spit. You should cook the meat for around 2 hours or until the temperature inside has reached 145 degrees Fahrenheit.

3. Whilst the meat is cooking taking the rest of the sauce, which you marinated the meat in originally and pour into a saucepan. Now heat it up until it starts to boil, and then cook for 5 minutes so it becomes reduced. You will then use this sauce for basting the meat whilst it is cooking. It is important that you baste the meat regularly during the last hour of cooking.

Barbecue Cookbook

Once the time for cooking has elapsed remove from heat and allow to stand for 15 minutes before you then slice and serve. Remember to keep the meat covered whilst it is resting.

RECIPE 20 – BARBECUED RIB EYE STEAK

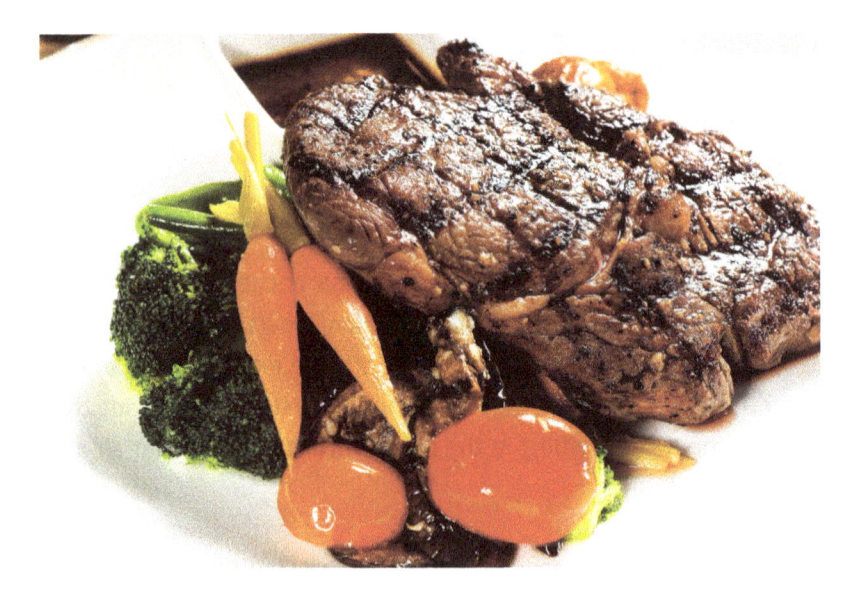

Although the ingredients used to make this meal are quite sweet the fat in the meat and bacon helps to counteract it.

Ingredients

280gram Marbled Rib Eye Steak

2 Teaspoons Garlic Powder

1 Teaspoon Salt

1 Teaspoon Freshly Ground Black Pepper

700ml Cola Flavored Drink

Samantha Michaels

950ml Barbecue Sauce

8 Slices Bacon

Instructions

1. Score the steaks on both sides using a sharp knife so that a diamond pattern is formed. Also make cuts into the fatty areas of the steak with the tip of the knife. Now sprinkle the steak with a small amount of the garlic powder, salt and pepper before then rubbing it into the scores you made previously. Do this to both sides of the steak.

2. Now place the steak into a shallow dish and pour over them the cola flavoured drink, cover and leave in the refrigerator to marinate for 4 hours. You should turn the steaks over every hour. Also during the last hour of marinating you should now cover the steak in a thin layer of the barbecue sauce.

3. After the steaks have marinated for 4 hours they are now ready to cook they should be cooked on the barbecue over a high heat. However before you place them on the grill make sure that it has been lightly oiled. Now cook on each side for about 4 minutes or until burnt.

4. Once this has been done either reduce the heat by turning the burners down or by moving the steak to a cooler part of the barbecue. Once you have moved the heat has been reduced place on top the bacon strips close the lid and then cook each side for 10 minutes. During the last few minutes of cooking again spread over a thin layer of barbecue sauce. Cooking until the sauce has become dried out and created a glazed effect to the meat.

CHAPTER 2- CHICKEN RECIPES

RECIPE 1 – ROTISSERIE CHICKEN

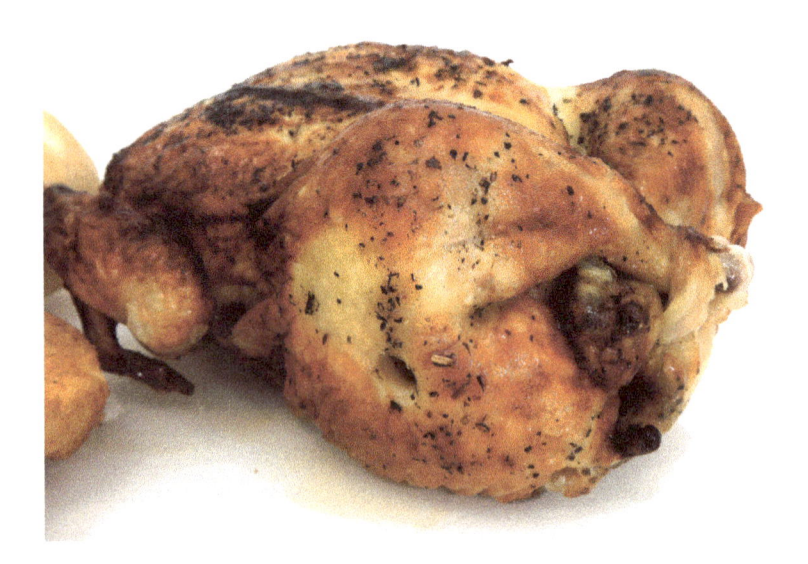

A very quick and easy meal to prepare and then cook on the barbecue. You can either serve it as the main part of the meal or as a starter.

Ingredients

1.36 Kg Whole Chicken

57gram Butter (Melted)

1 Tablespoon Salt

1 Tablespoon Paprika

¼ Tablespoon Ground Black Pepper

Instructions

1. Season the inside of the chicken using a pinch of salt. Then spear it with the rotisserie skewer before then placing on your preheated barbecue. Make sure that the heat is as hot as possible and then allow the chicken to cook for 10 minutes.

2. Whilst the chicken is cooking in a bowl mix together the melted butter, salt, paprika and pepper. Once the mixture is ready and the 10 minutes have elapsed reduce the heat and baste the chicken with the mixture you have just prepared.

3. Once all the chicken has been basted you can close the lid and cook the chicken for 1 to 1 ½ hours. Whilst it is cooking don't forget to regularly baste it with the mixture as this will help to prevent the meat from drying out. You know when the meat is ready when the juices run clear after inserting a skewer into the thickest part of the chicken body or when you insert a meat thermometer the internal temperature of the chicken has reached 180 degrees Fahrenheit.

4. After the meat has cooked you now remove it from the barbecue and allow it to rest for 10 to 15 minutes before then carving it up and serving. Whilst it is resting make sure that you keep the meat covered up.

RECIPE 2 – SHISH TAOUK GRILLED CHICKEN

Bored with your chicken kebabs always tasting the same, then give this particular recipe a whirl.

Barbecue Cookbook

Ingredients

907gram Chicken Breast (Cut Into 2 Inch Pieces)

2 Onions (Cut Into Large Chunks)

1 Large Green Bell Pepper (Cut Into Large Chunks And Seeds Removed)

60ml Fresh Lemon Juice

60ml Vegetable Oil

180ml Plain Yogurt

4 Cloves Garlic (Minced)

2 Teaspoons Tomato Paste

1 ½ Teaspoons Salt

1 Teaspoon Dried Oregano

¼ Teaspoon Ground Black Pepper

¼ Teaspoon Ground All Spice

¼ Teaspoon Ground Cinnamon

¼ Teaspoon Ground Cardamom

229gram Freshly Chopped Flat Leaf Parsley

Instructions

1. In a bowl whisk together the lemon juice, oil, yogurt, garlic, tomato paste, oregano, all spice, cinnamon, cardamom, oregano, pepper and salt. Then add the chicken and toss it through the mixture to make sure that all pieces are well coated. Then transfer to a large plastic bag (resealable kind is best) and place in the refrigerator for 4 hours.

2. Whilst you are threading the chicken, onions and bell pepper on to skewers start up the barbecue so it has reached the required temperature to cook these chicken kebabs. It is important that you cook the chicken over a medium to high heat for 5 minutes on each side. The exterior of the meat should be golden in color, whilst when you make an insertion in to the meat it should look white inside. Once they have been cooked through properly remove kebabs from heat then sprinkle over some of the flat leaf parsley before serving.

RECIPE 3 – GRILLED BUTTER CHICKEN

This particular recipe originally comes from India and is best made using a whole, which you or your butcher then cut up into pieces. The spices really help to make this dish much more flavorsome.

Ingredients

1.3 to 1.8 kg Whole Chicken (Cut Into Quarters And Skin Removed)

114gram of Pureed Onion

120ml Plain Yogurt

120ml Melted Butter or Clarified Butter (Ghee)

4 to 5 Cloves of Garlic (Minced)

1 Serrano Chili (Seeds Removed And Minced)

2 ½ Tablespoons Ground Ginger

1 Tablespoon Ground Coriander Seeds

1 Tablespoon Oil

1 ½ Teaspoons Salt

Instructions

1. Combine together the onion, yogurt, garlic, chili, ginger, coriander, oil and salt in a bowl. When combined together thoroughly now pour of the chicken pieces that have been placed in a shallow glass bowl. Now cover the chicken and allow it to marinate in the sauce for between 8 and 12 hours.

2. Next remove the chicken from the refrigerator and let it stand for 20 to 30 minutes. Whilst this is happening take half of the butter and melt it in saucepan and let it cook for 3 to 5 minutes.

3. Whilst the chicken is coming back up to room temperature turn on the barbecue so that you are able to then grill the meat on it at a medium to high heat. Make sure that the grill on which you place the meat has been lightly oiled first and then cook each piece of chicken for 25 to 30 minutes. You must make sure that you turn the chicken over regularly and baste it with the melted butter often. Once the chicken has cooked through remove from the grill. Now place on to a clean plate and pour over the rest of the butter.

Recipe 4 – Blackened Chicken

This particular recipe packs quite a punch. You will find that there is not only enough sauce for basting the chicken as it cooks but also to use as a dipping sauce as well.

Ingredients

4 Boneless And Skinless Chicken Breasts Halved

1 Tablespoon Paprika

4 Teaspoons Sugar (Divided)

1 ½ Teaspoons Salt

1 Teaspoon Garlic Powder

1 Teaspoon Dried Thyme

1 Teaspoon Lemon Pepper Seasoning

1 Teaspoon Cayenne Pepper

1 ½ Teaspoons Pepper (Divided)

320ml Mayonnaise

2 Tablespoons Water

2 Tablespoons Cider Vinegar

Instructions

1. In a small bowl place the paprika, 1 teaspoon sugar, 1 teaspoon salt, the garlic powder, lemon pepper, thyme, cayenne pepper, and

½ to 1 teaspoon of pepper. Mix well together then sprinkle over all sides of the chicken and set the meat to one side.

2. In another bowl you place the mayonnaise, water, vinegar and the rest of the sugar, salt and pepper. Once all ingredients have been combined together you put around 240ml of this to one side, which you place in the refrigerator to chill. The rest of the mixture is what you will be basting the chicken in.

3. To cook the chicken place over indirect medium heat on the barbecue. Remember to oil the grill first to ensure that the chicken doesn't stick to it then cook on each side for 4 to 6 minutes or until the juices that are released by the chicken as it cooks run clear. Don't forget as you are cooking the chicken on the grill to baste it regularly with the sauce made using the mayonnaise. After cooking serve with the sauce in the refrigerator.

Recipe 5 – Grilled Herb Chicken Burgers

As well as these burgers being low in fat they also taste extremely delicious. You will know if the burgers aren't cooked properly because they will be soft to the touch.

Ingredients

450gram Ground Chicken Breast

1 Small Carrot (Grated)

2 Green Onions (Minced)

2 Cloves Garlic (Minced)

1 Teaspoon Dried Parsley

Samantha Michaels

1 Teaspoon Dried Basil

¼ Teaspoon Salt

¼ Teaspoon Freshly Ground Black Pepper

Instructions

1. Into a large mixing bowl put the ground chicken meat, the carrot, onions, garlic, herbs, salt and pepper. Mix thoroughly together. It is best if you use your hands to do this. Whilst you are mixing these ingredients together then you should have the barbecue turned on or you should have lit the charcoal. So by the time the burgers are made you can then start cooking them.

2. After mixing the ingredients together you should make between 4 and 6 burgers from it. Before you cook them however place them on a sheet of wax paper and let them rest in the refrigerator for a few minutes.

3. Once the barbecue has heated up you must first lightly oil the grill before then placing the burgers on to it. To make sure that the chicken is cooked properly they should remain on the grill for between 12 and 15 minutes. It is important that during this time you turn them over at least once. You will know when they are cooked through, as the juices running out of them will run clear.

RECIPE 6 – GRILLED CHICKEN WING WITH SWEET RED CHILI & PEACH GLAZE

The adding of the peaches into the marinade helps to counteract some of the heat from the chilies.

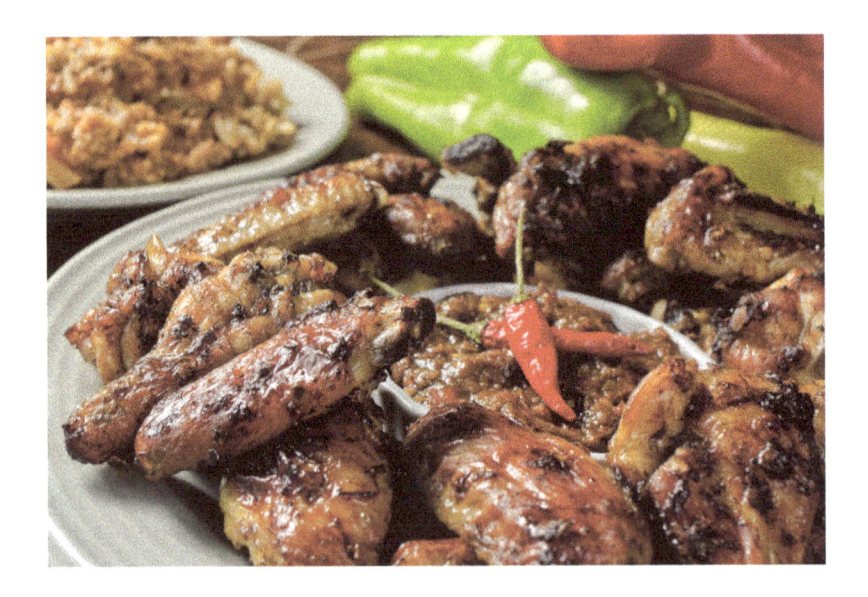

Ingredients

1.13Kg Chicken Wings

350ml Jar Of Peach Jam

240ml Thai Sweet Red Chili Sauce

1 Teaspoon Fresh Lime Juice

1 Tablespoon Fresh Cilantro (Minced)

Instructions

1. In a bowl mix together the peach jam, the chili sauce, the lime juice and cilantro. Take half of this mixture and pour into a bowl, as you will use this a dipping sauce to serve with the cooked chicken wings.

2. After your barbecue has reached the right temperature and you have sprayed the grill with oil to prevent the chicken wings from sticking place them on it. Grill the wings for between 20 and 25 minutes, remembering to turn them over frequently to ensure that they are cooked through evenly.

3. Only when the juices are running clear from the chickens can you then apply the remaining half of the sauce to glaze them. After applying the glaze make sure that you cook them for a further 3 to 5 minutes. Again you need to turn them over once during this time to make sure that they are well coated with the glaze.

RECIPE 7 – GRILLED CHICKEN KOFTAS

You can either eat these by themselves or you can use them as a filling for a sandwich or in pitta bread. If you are going to put them into pitta bread then warm the bread through first by placing it on the edge of the barbecue away from the direct heat source for a minute, turning them over after 30 seconds.

Ingredients

450gram Ground Chicken Breast

229gram Bread Crumbs

1 Egg (Lightly Beaten)

2 Cloves Garlic (Minced)

1 Tablespoon Cilantro (Finely Chopped)

1 Teaspoon Hot Sauce

1 Teaspoon Salt

¼ Teaspoon Freshly Ground Black Pepper

Instructions

1. In a large mixing bowl combine together the ground chicken breast, bread crumbs, egg, garlic, cilantro, hot sauce, salt and pepper. Then cover and allow to rest in the refrigerator as this will make it much easier to then form the Koftas (sausage shape patties), which you form around a metal skewer.

2. As soon as you have formed the Koftas around the skewer they are now ready to cook. Place them about 3 inches above the barbecue and allow them to cook for around 10 minutes. During this time make sure that you turn them frequently to ensure that they don't burn and that the meat cooks evenly. As soon as they are cooked you can then serve them.

Recipe 8 – Thai Grilled Chicken With A Chili Dipping Sauce

You will find this recipe quite refreshing and with the dipping sauce it really adds a new element to the whole dish.

Ingredients

1.36Kg Chicken Breast (Cut Into Pieces)

120ml Coconut Milk

Samantha Michaels

2 Tablespoons Fish Sauce

2 Tablespoons Garlic (Minced)

2 Tablespoons Fresh Chopped Cilantro

1 Teaspoon Ground Turmeric

1 Teaspoon Curry Powder

½ Teaspoon White Pepper

Dipping Sauce

6 Tablespoons Rice Vinegar

4 Tablespoons Water

4 Tablespoons Sugar

½ Teaspoon Minced Birds Eye Chilli

1 Teaspoon Garlic (Minced)

¼ Teaspoon Salt

Instructions

1. In a shallow dish mix the coconut milk, fish sauce, garlic, cilantro, turmeric, curry powder and white pepper. Then when thoroughly combined add the chicken pieces and turn them over in the sauce so that they are completely coated. Cover and place in the refrigerator for 4 hours or overnight to let the chicken pieces marinate in the sauce.

Barbecue Cookbook

2. Whilst the chicken is marinating you can now make the sauce. To do this you place the vinegar, water, sugar, garlic, chili and salt in to a saucepan and bring this mixture to the boil. Now lower the heat and let the mixture simmer for about 5 minutes. It is important you stir the sauce from time to time to prevent it sticking to the base of the saucepan and burning. Remove from heat and allow to cool before placing into a serving bowl.

3. When cooking the chicken on the barbecue make sure that the grill has been lightly oiled first. Cook each piece of chicken for 10 minutes on each side or until the juices start to running out of them clear. Brush them with a little of the sauce you made earlier before serving, whilst the rest remains in the serving dish and which people can then dip the chicken wings into if they wish.

RECIPE 9 – CATALAN CHICKEN QUARTERS

This is a Spanish inspired recipe where not only does the smoke help to enhance the flavor of the chicken so does the thick tomato sauce.

Ingredients

4 Chicken Leg Quarters

1 Onion (Chopped)

172gram Chorizo (Spicy Sausage Chopped)

1 Can Whole Tomatoes (Drained And Chopped)

120ml Red Wine

Samantha Michaels

114gram Olives (Pitted And Chopped)

5 Cloves Of Garlic (Minced)

2 Tablespoons Olive Oil

1 Teaspoon Salt

½ Teaspoon Cumin

½ Teaspoon Cinnamon

¼ Teaspoon Cayenne Pepper

¼ Teaspoon Freshly Ground Black Pepper

Instructions

1. In a bowl combine together the salt, cumin, black pepper and cayenne pepper and rub over the surface of the chicken, making sure you get as much of this rub under the skin of the chicken as well.

2. Allow the chicken to rest in the refrigerator for a while (covered) whilst you start preparing the sauce to go with them. To make the sauce sauté the onions and garlic in the olive oil before adding the sausage, tomatoes and red wine. Allow this to simmer on a low heat whilst you are then cooking the chicken quarters on the barbecue. You should cook the chicken quarters until the juice runs clear from them, remembering to turn them over often to prevent the skin from burning.

3. Whilst the chicken is cooking you should now add the olives to the sauce and continue simmering it for a further 20 minutes.

4. To serve simply place one of the chicken quarters on to a plate and then pour over some of the sauce.

Recipe 10 – Thai Chicken Satay

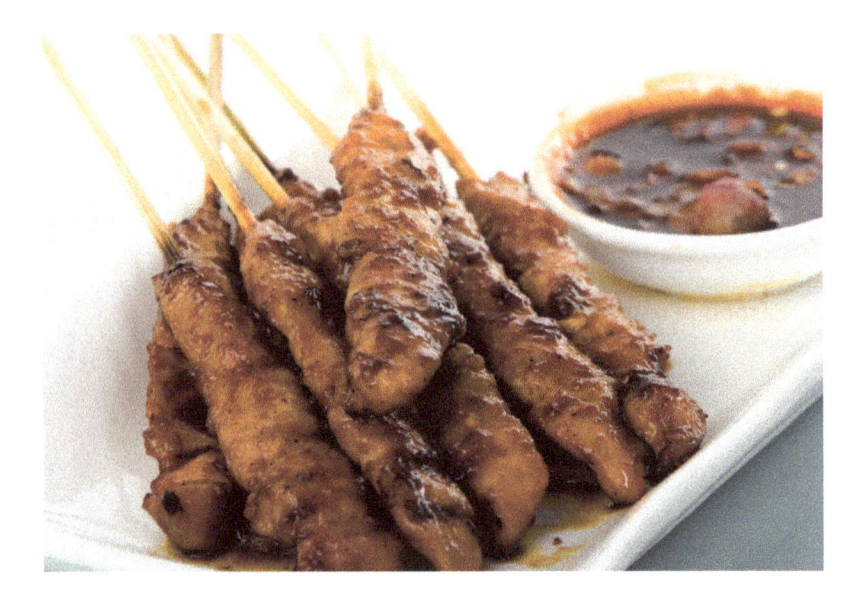

Unfortunately this is a recipe you shouldn't be trying if you or someone you know is allergic to peanuts.

Ingredients

907gram Chicken Breasts Without The Skin (Cut Into Strips)

2 Tablespoons Vegetable Oil

2 Tablespoons Soy Sauce

2 Teaspoons Tamarind Paste

1 Stalk Lemon Grass (Chopped)

Samantha Michaels

2 Cloves Garlic (Crushed)

1 Teaspoon Ground Cumin

1 Teaspoon Ground Coriander

1 Tablespoon Fresh Lime Juice

1 Teaspoon Muscovado Sugar

½ Teaspoon Chili Powder

Sauce

2 Tablespoons Peanut Butter (Crunchy)

2 Tablespoons Peanuts (Chopped)

1 Can Coconut Milk

2 Teaspoon Red Thai Curry Paste

1 Tablespoon Fish Sauce

1 Teaspoon Tomato Paste

1 Tablespoon Brown Sugar

Instructions

1. You first need to make up the sauce in which the chicken pieces will be marinated. To do it get a large bowl and into place the vegetable oil, soy sauce, tamarind paste, lemon grass, garlic, cumin, coriander, lime juice, sugar and chili powder. Make sure that you

combine these ingredients well before adding the chicken and stir round until you know all the chicken pieces have been coated in the marinade. Cover the bowl and place in the refrigerator for one hour.

2. Whilst the chicken is marinating you can make the satay (peanut) sauce. To do this into a small saucepan put the peanut butter, peanuts, coconut milk, red Thai curry paste, fish sauce, tomato paste and sugar. Cook the ingredients on a medium to low heat, making sure that you stir it frequently and until it looks smooth. It is important that you keep the sauce warm after it has been made so turn the heat down as low as possible and cover.

3. To cook the chicken pieces you first need to thread them onto skewers and when this is turn place them on to the lightly oiled barbecue grill and allow them to cook on each side for around 3 to 5 minutes. Once the chicken is thoroughly cooked remove from the heat and either pour the satay sauce over them or provide it in a bowl which guests can then dip their chicken kebabs if they wish.

RECIPE 11 – BARBECUE CHICKEN BREASTS

You will find that this particular recipe becomes one that you will use time and time again. When cooked correctly the exterior of the chicken becomes crispy whilst the interior remains moist.

Ingredients

4 x 250gram Skinless Chicken Breasts

Zest Of 1 Orange

1 Dried Chili

1 ½ Teaspoons (Heaped) Smoked Paprika

1 ½ Teaspoons Dijon or English Mustard

3 Tablespoons Honey

3 Tablespoons Tomato Ketchup

1 Teaspoon Olive Oil

1/16 Teaspoon Sea Salt

Freshly Ground Black Pepper To Taste

Instructions

1. Into a bowl put the finely grated zest of the orange, along with the dried chili (crumbled), the paprika, mustard, honey, tomato ketchup and the olive oil. Then after combining all these ingredients together add a pinch of salt along with some pepper then stir again.

2. Take out a couple of spoonfuls of the mixture made and put to one side. To the rest of the marinade in the bowl you add the chicken breasts. Turn them over so that they are completed coated by the marinade made and cover with plastic wrap before leaving to one side for 5 to 10 minutes.

3. Once the barbecue has heated up correctly you need to put the chicken on the grill but before you do make sure that you lightly oil it. When you place them on the grill make sure that the heat underneath isn't too high. If you notice the outer part of the chicken is starting to char quickly then move them over to a cooler part of the barbecue and reduce the heat if possible. You should be aiming to cook the chickens on each side for about 5 minutes, turning them every minute and basting them with some more of the marinade left in the bowl. You should only remove them from

the heat when they have turned a golden brown and are cooked all the way through.

The best way of testing to see that they are cooked all the way through is to push a skewer in to. If the juices that flow out are clear then you know the chicken is properly cooked. Remove from heat, then place on clean plates and spoon some of the sauce that you put aside earlier over them.

Recipe 12 – Spicy Plum Chicken Thighs

The plum sauce that coats the chicken thighs creates a slightly sweeter tasting barbecue sauce. It is important that you don't cook the thighs over too high a heat otherwise this could result in the sauce burning.

Ingredients

8 Chicken Thighs (Skin On And Bone In)

Salt and Freshly Ground Black Pepper

Plum Sauce

2 Tablespoons Peanut Oil

1 Small Coarsely Chopped Onion

4 Cloves Garlic (Coarsely Chopped)

1 Tablespoon Fresh Coarsely Chopped Ginger

1 Coarsely Chopped Thai Chili

¼ Teaspoon Ground Cinnamon

¼ Teaspoon Ground Cloves

680gram Red or Purple Plums (Pitted and Coarsely Chopped)

60ml Honey

60ml Soy Sauce

2 Tablespoons Fresh Lime Juice

1 Tablespoon Granulated Sugar

Instructions

1. Before you do anything else you need to make the plum sauce. To do this in a medium size saucepan place the oil and heat it up. When it is hot enough add the onions and garlic and cook until they are soft. Then add to these the ginger, cinnamon, Thai chili and cloves and cook for 2 minutes. Now you need to add the rest of the ingredients listed above and cook until the plums have softened and the sauce has started to thicken. Then place the mixture into a food processor or blender and mix them until smooth. Pour into a bowl and allow to cool.

2. After making the sauce you need to heat the barbecue up to a medium low indirect heat for cooking the chicken thighs. Just before you place the chicken thighs on to the grill lightly oil it first and season the thighs with salt and pepper. Cook on either side until they turn a light golden brown between 1 and 5 minutes.

3. Now brush one side of the chicken with the plum sauce made earlier and turn the thighs over and continue cooking for 3 to 4 minutes. Once this time has elapsed brush the sides of the thighs facing you with more sauce and again turn them over to cook for another 3 to 4 minutes. You should continue turning and basting

the thighs with the plum sauce until they are cooked through. You will find that they will be cooked through properly after 15 to 20 minutes. However if you are unsure just insert a skewer in to the thickest part of the thigh. If you notice the juices running out are clear then the chicken is cooked.

4. Please don't forget to keep the thighs at a good height above the heat to prevent them and the sauce from burning.

RECIPE 13 – MAPLE BARBECUED CHICKEN

You will find that the sweet flavor of the maple helps to really make this dish stand out and may have guests at your barbecue asking for seconds. To obtain the best results possible use a good quality syrup. Of course if you want to give this recipe a little kick then add some hot chili sauce as well.

Ingredients

4 Skinless Chicken Thighs

3 Tablespoons Maple Syrup

3 Tablespoons Hot Chili Sauce (Optional)

1 Tablespoon Cider Vinegar

1 Tablespoon Canola Oil

2 Teaspoon Dijon Mustard

Salt

Freshly Ground Pepper

Samantha Michaels

Instructions

1. Whilst the barbecue is heating up in a saucepan combine together the maple syrup, cider vinegar and mustard. Plus of course the hot chili sauce if you are looking to give this recipe an extra kick. After mixing the ingredients together place saucepan on a medium heat and let the mixture simmer for 5 minutes.

2. Next you need to brush the chicken with the oil before then sprinkling on some salt and pepper to season. Then place them on to the grill and cook for between 10 and 15 minutes. As you cook them turn them regularly and each time that you turn them brush a generous amount of the sauce over them. Once cooked place on a clean plate and serve immediately. Any sauce left over can either be poured over the chicken thighs or placed a bowl, which the thighs can then be dipped into.

Recipe 14 – Spatchcock Barbecue Chicken

It is best if you get your butcher to cut the chicken up for doing this recipe.

Ingredients

1.3kg Spatchcock Chicken

3 Tablespoon Olive Oil

1 Teaspoon Paprika

1 Garlic Clove Crushed

Juice and Zest Of 1 Lemon

A Little Water or Beer to Taste

Salt

Freshly Ground Pepper

2 Lemons Quartered

Instructions

1. Whilst the barbecue is heating up in a bowl mix together the oil, garlic, paprika, lemon zest, salt and pepper. Once all these ingredients have been mixed together you brush it all over the skin of the chicken before then placing it covered in the fridge for 30 minutes to allow it to marinate.

2. When it comes to cooking the chicken on the barbecue you should cook it initially for 5 minutes on each side in the middle of the barbecue. Then move over to the side so that the heat cooking it is much gentler. It is important whilst the chicken is cooking that you turn it regularly and baste in between each turn with either beer or water. The best way of determining when the chicken is cooked through is to pierce between the thigh and breast bone with a sharp knife. When you do the flesh should feel firm and should look white.

You should be cooking each side of the chicken for between 20 and 30 minutes. Plus place something over the top, as the steam produced will help the chicken to cook through.

3. Once the chicken has cooked you now need to remove it from the heat and leave it to rest. Make sure that you cover it with foil and leave it to rest for around 10 to 15 minutes. Once this time has passed cut it up into pieces and drizzle some lemon juice, oil, salt,

pepper and paprika over them. Then serve on a fresh plate with the lemon quarters.

RECIPE 15 – CHICKEN TIKKA SKEWERS

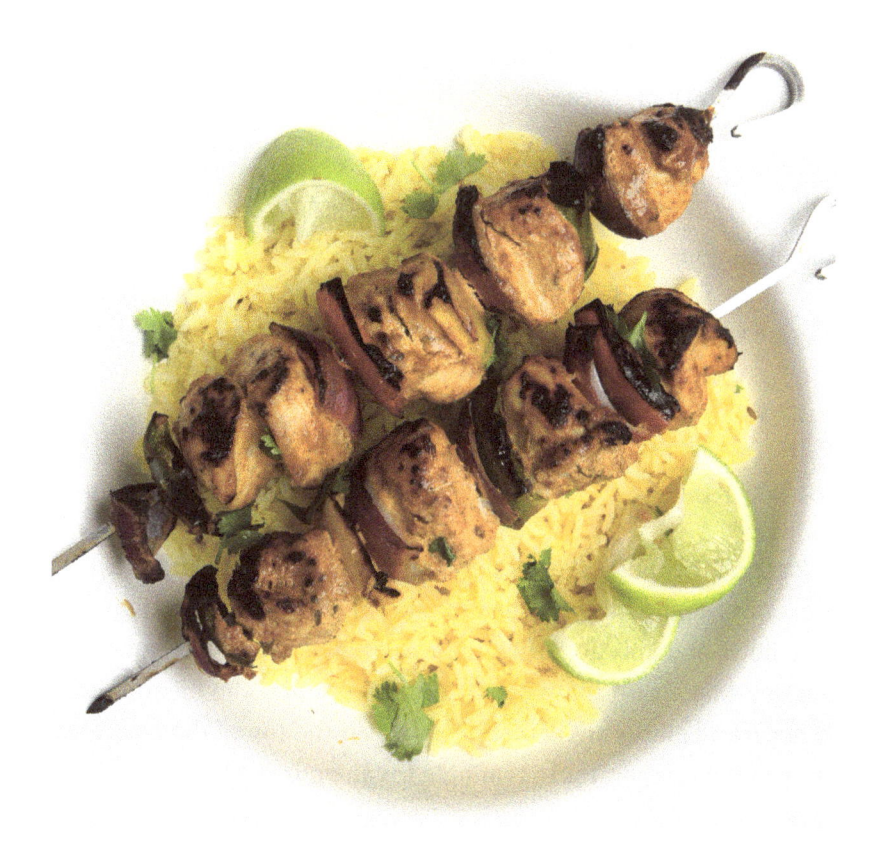

As well as being a quick and easy dish to prepare for your barbecue this summer, this particular recipe is also low in calories.

Ingredients

4 Skinless Boneless Chicken Breasts Cut Into Cubes

150gram Low Fat Natural Yogurt

Barbecue Cookbook

2 Tablespoon Hot Curry Paste

250gram Cherry Tomatoes

4 Wholemeal Chapattis

½ Cucumber Cut In Half Lengthways, Deseeded and then Sliced

1 Red Onion Thinly Sliced

Handful Coriander Leaves Chopped

Juice 1 Lemon

50gram Lamb's Lettuce or Pea Shoots

Instructions

1. Place the wooden skewers (8 in all) in some water in a bowl to soak. After doing this you need to place the yogurt and curry paste in a bowl and mix together then to this you add the cubes of chicken. Make sure that you stir the chicken into the mixture well to ensure all pieces are coated. Now cover the top of the bowl and place in the refrigerator to marinate for an hour or so.

2. Next in another bowl place the cucumber, red onion, coriander and lemon and toss them altogether. Again place this bowl in the refrigerator (covered over) and leave there until you are ready to serve the chicken.

3. Whilst the barbecue is heated up now you need to start preparing the skewers. You must make sure that you shake off any excess marinade before then threading the pieces of chicken on to the skewers. After threading on a piece of chicken now thread on a cherry tomato and do this until all skewers have been used.

4. Once the Chicken Tikka skewers are ready and the barbecue has heated up you are now ready to start cooking. You should keep the skewers on the barbecue for between 15 and 20 minutes, making sure that you turn them regularly so that they get cooked through and become a nice brown color.

5. When it comes to serving the skewers place them to one side on a clean plate to rest for a few minutes whilst you prepare the salad. Into the salad before serving mix the lettuce and pea shoots and divide this equally between four plates and on top of which you then place two of the skewers. Serve them with chapattis that have been warmed through on the barbecue. The best way to warm the chapattis on the barbecue is to wrap them in some aluminum foil.

RECIPE 16 – SWEET & SPICY WINGS WITH SUMMER COLESLAW

Just like many other recipes in this book this is one that is very quick and easy to make and will certainly help to add a little spice to your barbecue this summer.

Ingredients

1kg Chicken Wings

4 Tablespoon Curry Paste (Tikka would be wonderful)

3 Tablespoon Mango Chutney

200g Sliced Radishes

1 Cucumber Halved Lengthways And Sliced

1 Small Bunch Roughly Chopped Mint

Juice Of 1 Lemon

Instructions

1. Start getting the barbecue heated up. Now in to a large bowl place the curry paste and 2 tablespoons of the mango chutney with a little salt and pepper to season, then stir well.

2. Place the chicken wings in the mixture and toss around so that they are all well coated and then leave to marinate for a short while.

3. Now place on to the barbecue griddle making sure that the surface has been lightly oiled first to prevent the chicken sticking to it. Now cook for between 40 and 45 minutes, turning occasionally until all sides are golden brown and the wings are cooked through. The quickest way to determine if the wings have been cooked through is to stick a skewer into the thickest part and when removed do the juices run clear.

4. Finally just before you are about to serve the chicken wings in another bowl place the radishes, cucumber, mint, the rest of the mango chutney and the lemon juice and stir thoroughly. Now place the chicken wings on a clean plate and then beside it place the freshly made coleslaw.

RECIPE 17 – STICKY CHICKEN DRUMSTICKS

This isn't only a recipe that kids will enjoy eating so will many adults, especially those with somewhat of a sweet tooth.

Ingredients

8 Chicken Drumsticks

2 Tablespoon Soy Sauce

1 Tablespoon Honey

1 Tablespoon Olive Oil

1 Tablespoon Tomato Puree

1 Tablespoon Dijon Mustard

Instructions

1. You need to make 3 slashes into each chicken drumstick as this will then help the meat to absorb quite a bit of the marinade you are about to make. Then place the drumsticks into a shallow dish.

2. To make the marinade you need to place the soy sauce, honey, olive oil, mustard and tomato puree into a bowl and whisk together thoroughly. Once all these ingredients have been combined pour some over the drumsticks before turning them over and pouring the remainder of the marinade over them. Once this has been done you must place them in the refrigerator overnight (remembering to cover them).

3. Whilst the barbecue is heating up ready for you to cook the drumsticks remove them from the refrigerator and allow them to come up to room temperature. When the barbecue is heated up sufficiently you can now place the drumsticks on to the grill. Although there is oil in the marinade don't forget to brush some

Barbecue Cookbook

over the grill to prevent the chicken drumsticks from sticking to them.

4. It is important that you cook these for around 35 minutes or until the juice inside them starts to run clear. Also it is important to remember to turn them over regularly to prevent the exterior from becoming burnt and also to ensure that they cook right through. Once they are cooked now place them on a clean plate and serve to your waiting guests.

RECIPE 18 – JERK CHICKEN KEBABS AND MANGO SALSA

The inclusion of a mango salsa with these kebabs helps to take some of the kick out of the spices used in making the Jerk Chicken.

Ingredients

Jerk Chicken

4 Skinless Chicken Breasts Cut Into Chunks

2 Teaspoon Jerk Seasoning

1 Tablespoon Olive Oil

Juice of 1 Lime

1 Large Yellow Pepper Cut Into 2cm Cubes

Samantha Michaels

Mango Salsa

320g Mango Diced

1 Large Red Pepper Deseeded and Diced

Bunch Spring Onions Finely Chopped

1 Red Chili Chopped (This Is Optional)

Instructions

1. In a bowl place the jerk seasoning, olive oil and lime juice and then mix thoroughly together. A whisk would be best to do this. Then once all these ingredients have been thoroughly combined toss the chunks of chicken in it and place in the refrigerator for at least 20 minutes. However if you really want the meat to absorb as much of the marinade as possible then it is best to leave it in the refrigerator for at least 24 hours.

2. Once the meat has time to marinade you are now ready to start cooking it. But whilst the barbecue is heating up you can now start making the salsa. To do this you simply place all the ingredients mentioned above in a bowl and stir together. Add a little salt and pepper to season then place in the refrigerator until you are ready to serve it with the kebabs.

3. To make the kebabs you need some wooden skewers, which have been left in some water for at least 30 minutes. Remember doing this will prevent them from burning. Now on to each skewer you thread a piece of chicken followed by a piece of the yellow pepper. You should be aiming to put on each of the 8 skewers 3 pieces of meat and 3 pieces of pepper.

4. Once the kebabs have been made and the barbecue is hot enough you can start cooking them. Each side of the kebab should be cooked for around 8 minutes. This will not only ensure that they are cooked through but also helps to create a little charring on them. Once they are cooked place two kebabs on a plate and add some salsa

Recipe 19 – Chicken & Chorizo Kebabs With Chimichurri

This really is something different and the chorizo along with the Chimichurri helps to provide a little bit of spice to these kebabs.

Ingredients

250g Chicken Breast Cut Into Chunks

250g Chorizo Cut Into Chunks

Olive Oil For Brushing The Kebabs

Chimichurri

4 Tablespoon Freshly Chopped Parsley

1 Red Chili Chopped

1 Garlic Clove Chopped

2 Teaspoon Dried Oregano

2 Teaspoon Smoked Paprika

5 Tablespoon Olive Oil

2 Tablespoon Red Wine Vinegar

Instructions

1. On to several skewers you need to place chunks of the chicken and chorizo sausage and then lightly season with some salt and pepper before then brushing with some olive oil before placing on to the barbecue. It is important that whilst cooking these for around 10 minutes you turn them regularly to prevent them from becoming burnt.

2. Whilst the kebabs are cooking you can now make the Chimichurri sauce. This is very simple to do simply place all the ingredients above in a bowl and then whisk thoroughly. By the time you have done this the kebabs should have cooked and will be ready to serve. Simply place two kebabs on each clean plate and serve a small bowl of the Chimichurri beside them.

RECIPE 20 – BARBECUED CHICKEN BURGERS

If you are having a last minute barbecue one summer evening you will be able to serve these very quickly to your family and friends.

Ingredients

4 Skinless Chicken Breasts

4 Tablespoon Tomato Ketchup

4 Tablespoon Brown Sauce

2 Teaspoon Clear Honey

2 Garlic Cloves Crushed

Splash Of Chili Sauce (Optional)

Instructions

1. In a large bowl combine together the tomato ketchup, brown sauce, honey and garlic cloves. It is at this time you also add the chili sauce if you wish this will give this sweet recipe a little kick. Once this has been done put take some of the mixture out as this you can then use as a sauce that people can put on to the chicken burgers after they have cooked.

2. Next you need to cut halfway into the thickest part of the chicken breast and then open it up in the same way you would a book. You should flatten the breasts down slightly using the palm of your hand then place them in the bowl with the marinade and toss to ensure all parts of the breast are coated with it. Now place in the refrigerator for around 20 minutes (remembering to cover the breasts over).

3. Whilst the barbecue is heating up you now need to remove the chicken from the refrigerator to bring it back up to room temperature. Once the barbecue is heated up sufficiently you can now place the chicken breasts on the grill, remembering to brush it lightly with oil first. You should cook each chicken breast for around 10 minutes or until they are cooked through. Also whilst cooking the breasts remember to turn them over regularly to help

the marinade to become sticky and also to help prevent the meat from burning.

4. Once they are cooked you can place them in buns with slices of bacon (cooked) and some lettuce and slices of tomato and onion. Plus don't forget to add a dollop of the sauce you put to one side earlier.

Chapter 3 - Pork Recipes

Recipe 1 – Pork Kebabs And Mushrooms

You will find that not only do these kebabs take very little time to prepare but also take very little time to cook, but make a great addition to any barbecue.

Ingredients

450gram Pork Fillet Cut Into 1 Inch Chunks

4 Tablespoon Olive Oil

2 Garlic Cloves Crushed

24 Button Mushrooms

24 Fresh Sage Leaves

Salt

Freshly Ground Black Pepper

Instructions

1. The first thing you need to do if you are going to be using wooden skewers for making the kebabs is to soak them in some water for at least half an hour. This will then help to ensure that they don't burn when placed on the barbecue.

2. Now you need to prepare the pork. To do this you need to place in a bowl the olive oil, garlic, salt and pepper and mix together

thoroughly. Once this has been done now you need to put the chunks of pork in to the mixture and toss them around thoroughly so each piece of meat is thoroughly coated. Then you can leave the meat in the refrigerator or to one side for 20 minutes or more. It is best to let the meat stay in the sauce for at least 20 minutes to help it absorb some of it.

3. Whilst the barbecue is heating up now you are ready to start making the kebabs on to each skewer thread pieces of pork with the mushrooms and sage leaves. Ideally you should thread on one piece of meat and then one mushroom and sage leave and continue doing this until all skewers have these ingredients on them.

4. Once the kebabs are ready you should cook them over a high heat on the barbecue for 15 to 20 minutes remembering to turn them often to prevent them from burning. Plus baste them regularly with any of the sauce that remains. As soon as the meat is cooked through then they are ready to serve.

RECIPE 2 – BARBECUED PORK STEAKS

This will really provide you with a very traditional barbecue recipe for that you can enjoy.

Ingredients

4 Pork Blade Steaks that are between 1 and 1 ¼ Inches Thick

120ml Bottle Barbecue Sauce

80ml Honey

Barbecue Cookbook

1 Tablespoon Worcestershire Sauce

1 Teaspoon Garlic Salt

½ Teaspoon Dijon Mustard

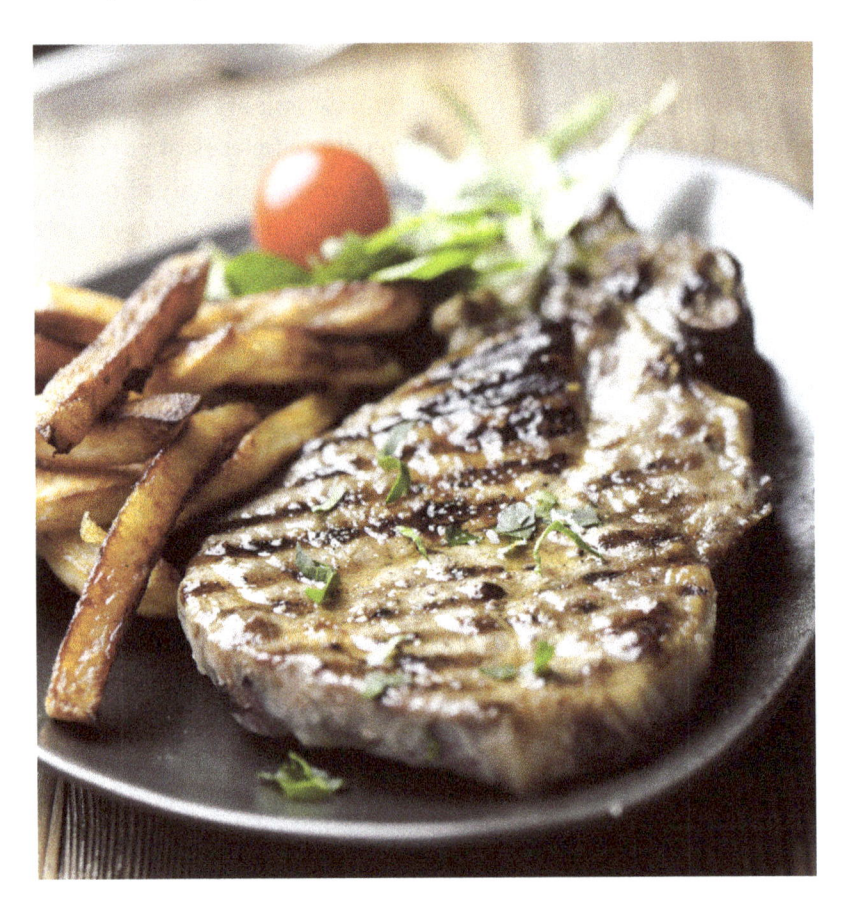

Instructions

1. In a bowl combine together the barbecue sauce, honey, Worcestershire sauce, garlic salt and mustard. This you will then use to baste the pork steaks as they cook.

2. To cook the pork steaks you need to place them on an oiled grill about 4 inches above the heat source. This will provide them with a medium heat to cook and will also ensure that they cook slowly so more of the moisture is retained.

3. You should cook each steak for around 8 minutes on each side before you then cook them for a further five minutes. But the last five minutes is when the pork should be brushed with the sauce. It is important that you turn the steaks over regularly during this last five minutes to ensure that they are both well coated in the sauce and to help it adhere to the surface of them.

4. Once the steaks are cooked place onto clean plates and serve with a crispy green salad and some nice crusty bread.

Recipe 3 – Barbecued Pork Kebabs

These have a more oriental flavor to them but taste just as wonderful as conventional barbecued pork kebabs do.

Ingredients

2 Kg Boneless Pork Loin Cut Into 1 ½ Inch Cubes

128gram White Sugar

240ml Soy Sauce

1 Onion Diced

5 Garlic Cloves Chopped

1 Teaspoon Ground Black Pepper

Instructions

1. Into a bowl place the sugar, soy sauce, onion, garlic and black pepper and whisk together well. Then to this you add the diced up

pork and toss to ensure that all pieces are thoroughly coated in the marinade.

2. Now cover the bowl over and place in the refrigerator for at least 2 hours. However if you really want the meat to taste even much sweeter then allow the pork to remain in the marinade overnight.

3. Whilst you are preparing the kebabs you should get the barbecue ready. Place the grill at a level so that the heat is very hot and make sure that it has been lightly oiled before you place the kebabs on it.

4. On to each wooden skewer, which has been soaking in water for 30 minutes, you thread on some of the pork. Once all the skewers have pork on them they are ready to cook. Ideally you should cook each side of the kebab for between 3 and 5 minutes or until the center of the meat is no longer pink. As soon as the kebabs have cooked you can serve them up to your guests with such accompaniments as coleslaw, rice or potato salad.

Recipe 4 – Honey Mustard Pork Chops

Although these are quite sweet the use of the vinegar, wine and mustard in the marinade helps to counteract some of this.

Ingredients

4 Pork Chops (3/4 Inch Thick Ones Are Best)

90ml Honey

3 Tablespoon Fresh Orange Juice

1 Tablespoon Cider Vinegar

1 Tablespoon White Wine

2 Teaspoon Worcestershire Sauce

2 Teaspoon Onion Powder

½ Teaspoon Dried Tarragon

3 Tablespoon Dijon Mustard

Instructions

1. Into a small bowl place the honey, orange, vinegar, wine, Worcestershire sauce, onion powder, tarragon and mustard and mix together. Now place to one side.

2. Next take the pork chops and make some cuts into the fatty edge of each one. This will then prevent the meat from actually curling whilst it is cooking on the barbecue. However make sure that you don't cut into the fat too far. Once this has been done place in a shallow dish and pour some of the marinade over them before then turning the chops over and pouring the rest of the marinade over them. Cover and place in the refrigerator for at least 2 hours.

3. Whilst the barbecue is heating up remove the chops from the refrigerator to allow them to come up to room temperature. Once the barbecue is hot enough and you have lightly oiled the grill you can place the chops on it. Cook each side of the chop for about 12 to 15 minutes and during this time turning them over at least 3 or 4 times. Each time you turn the chops over remember to brush on any of the marinade that is left over.

Once cooked you can now serve them on a clean plate with say a fresh green salad and a jacket potato.

Recipe 5 – Simple Grilled Pork Chops

The perfect recipe to use when you want to prepare something quick and simple to cook on the barbecue.

Ingredients

4 Pork Rib Chops About 1 Inch Thick

60ml Lemon Juice

3 Tablespoons Soy Sauce

1 Tablespoon Olive Oil

½ Teaspoon Brown Sugar

¼ Teaspoon Freshly Chopped Rosemary

Salt

Freshly Ground Black Pepper

Instructions

1. The first thing you need to do is make the marinade for the chops. To do this in a bowl place the lemon juice, soy sauce, olive oil, brown sugar, rosemary, salt and pepper. Then mix to ensure that they are combined together well.

2. Next you need to place the pork chops in a shallow dish or a resealable plastic bag and then pour over the chops the marinade made just now. Make sure that you toss the pork chops in this mix to ensure that all sides of them are coated in it. Once this has been done either cover the dish over or seal up the bag and place in the refrigerator for 30 minutes.

3. After the 30 minutes has elapsed remove the chops from the refrigerator and leave to one side to come up to room temperature. Also after taking the chops out of the refrigerator now is when you should be heating the barbecue up. As soon as the barbecue is ready you can now start cooking the chops.

4. The grill, which has been lightly oiled, should be placed quite close to the heat source as this will then help to sear the meat and ensure plenty of the meats juices are retained whilst you then cook them on a medium heat for 6 to 8 minutes. To reduce the heat you simply move the grill up away from the heat source. Also when cooking the chops remember to turn them over regularly to prevent them from burning.

As soon as the chops are cooked you should serve them immediately to your guests on a nice clean plate with say a jacket potato and coleslaw.

RECIPE 6 – BASIC BARBECUED PORK SPARE RIBS

No barbecue is complete without people having barbecued pork ribs served to them. If you have never tried cooking such food before this is one of the simplest recipes you can use.

Ingredients

1.36 Kg Pork Spare Ribs

240ml Ready Made Barbecue Sauce

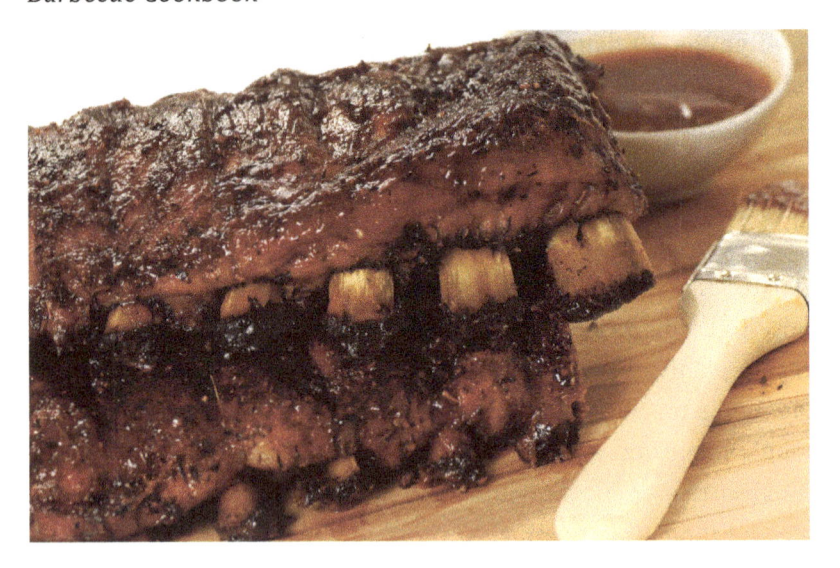

Instructions

1. Take the ribs and place them over a low heat on the barbecue and cook for between 1 and 1 ½ hours. You could of course cut down the cooking time if you wish by initially cooking them in the oven.

2. About 15 minutes before you then remove the pork spare ribs from the barbecue you now start to brush them with the barbecue sauce. It is important that during these last minutes of cooking is that you turn the ribs over and baste them with the sauce regularly. This will then help to ensure that all sides of the ribs get a good coating of the sauce and also will help to prevent the sauce from burning.

3. As soon as the ribs are cooked remove from the barbecue and cut up into portions that people will find easy to eat. Also it is a good idea to serve them with freshly made coleslaw and some crusty bread.

RECIPE 7 – SOUTHERN PULLED PORK

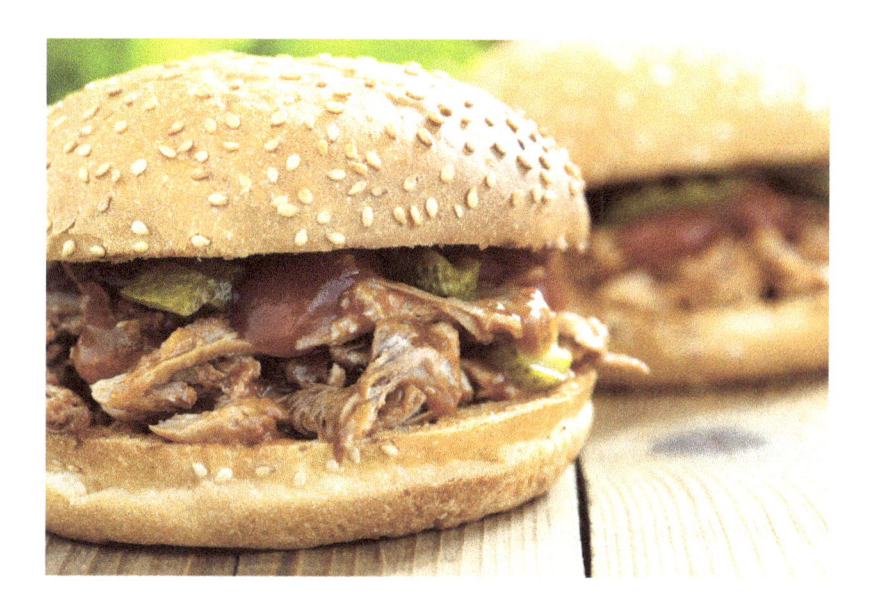

This is a very traditional recipe enjoyed in the southern parts of the USA. Once cooked traditionally the meat is then served on a bun and some coleslaw. Plus also gets served with lots of hot vinegar sauce.

Ingredients

1.8 to 2.2 Kg Pork Shoulder Roast

2 Tablespoons Paprika

1 Tablespoon Brown Sugar

1 Tablespoon Chili Powder

1 Tablespoon Ground Cumin

1 Tablespoon White Sugar

1 ½ Teaspoons Ground Black Pepper

2 Teaspoons Salt

1 Teaspoon Ground Red Pepper

Instructions

1. Into a bowl place all the spices to form a dry rub and then press it well into all the pork's surfaces.   Whilst you are doing this you should get the barbecue heated up ready for cooking.

2. As soon as the barbecue has heated and you have placed the grill high above the heat source you can now put the pork on to cook. When placed on the grill it will now require between 2.5 and 3 hours to cook. Whilst cooking it is important that you turn the meat regularly to prevent it from burning. Also to make sure that the meat is cooking properly insert a meat thermometer into the centre of it. The right temperature inside the meat, which will ensure it is cooked through, should be 170 degrees Fahrenheit.

3. After the cooking time has elapsed you now need to remove the pork from the barbecue and leave it to rest for around 10 minutes. Then it is ready to be shredded. You do this by using two forks to pull the meat apart and it is this action, which has given this recipe its name. As soon as you have done this place the meat on a clean plate and allow your guests to take a bun and pile it on it before adding some hot sauce if they want.

Recipe 8 – Grilled Pork Tenderloin Satay

If you are looking for a more healthy option to provide your guests with at your next barbecue this is a great recipe to consider trying.

However be aware that you shouldn't serve such food to any guests who may have a nut allergy.

Ingredients

450gram Pork Tenderloin

1 Small Chopped Onion

32gram Brown Sugar

60ml Water

3 Tablespoons Reduced Sodium Soy Sauce

2 Tablespoons Reduced Fat Creamy Peanut Butter

4 ½ Teaspoons Canola Oil

2 Garlic Cloves Minced

¼ Teaspoon Ground Ginger

Instructions

1. In a small saucepan put the onion, sugar, water, soy sauce, peanut butter, canola oil, garlic and ginger. Then over a medium heat bring these ingredients to a boil before turning the heat down so that they start simmering and leave uncovered for 10 to 12 minutes or until the sauce has started to thicken. To prevent the sauce from sticking to the base of the saucepan and burning you need to be stirring it regularly.

As soon as the sauce has become thick remove from heat and place about 120ml to one side.

2. Take the pork tenderloin and cut in half width wise before then cutting each half into thin strips than you then thread on to eight wooden or metal skewers. If you are using wooden skewers remember to soak them in water for ½ hour.

3. To cook place them on a lightly oiled grill on the barbecue over a medium to hot heat and cook on each side for 2 to 3 minutes. It is important whilst the kebabs are cooking that you baste them regularly with the sauce you made earlier. The meat will be cooked when it no longer looks pink.

To serve these kebabs simply place them on a clean plate along with the reserved sauce and allow guests to pick them up and then dip in the sauce.

RECIPE 9 – EASY TERIYAKI KEBABS

These particular pork kebabs can be made in a matter of minutes, as you will be using a ready prepared teriyaki marinade.

Ingredients

900gram Pork Tenderloin - Trimmed And Cut Into 1 Inch Cubes

240ml Ready Prepared Teriyaki Sauce

2 Tablespoons Vegetable Oil

1 20 Ounce Can Pineapple Chunks Drained

Samantha Michaels

500gram Cherry Tomatoes

2 Red or Green Bell Peppers – Cut Into 1 ½ Inch Pieces

Instructions

1. Piece the cubes of pork tenderloin so that the meat can absorb the sauce and oil you are using to marinate them in.

2. To make the marinade simply pour the sauce and oil into a bowl and whisk. However before pouring it over the pork make sure that you keep at least 2 tablespoons to one side in a separate bowl. Once poured over the meat cover and place in a refrigerator and leave for at least 1 hour. Whilst it is in the fridge make sure that you turn the meat occasionally this will then help to ensure that as much of the teriyaki sauce is absorbed by the meat.

3. After 1 hour remove the meat from the fridge then thread on to skewers. After each piece of meat thread on a piece of pineapple, a tomato and some pepper. Continue doing this until all ingredients have been used up. It is important that whilst you are doing this that the barbecue should be heating up.

4. To cook the kebabs you place them on the lightly oiled grill about 4 or 5 inches above the heat source and cook them on the barbecue for 15 minutes. It is important that when cooking these kebabs you turn them over frequently and brush with the marinade placed to one side earlier.

As soon as the kebabs are cooked served with a noodle or rice salad.

Barbecue Cookbook

Recipe 10 – Baby Back Barbecued Ribs

You can either start of by cooking these in the oven wrapped in aluminum foil or you can do the same on the barbecue. Then you finish them off by removing the foil and backing on the barbecue.

Ingredients

1.36Kg Baby Back Pork Ribs

1 Tablespoon Brown Sugar

1 Tablespoon Paprika

2 Teaspoons Garlic Powder

1 ½ Teaspoons Ground Black Pepper

120ml Water

350ml Ready Made Barbecue Sauce

Instructions

1. Before wrapping the baby back pork ribs in aluminum foil combine together the sugar, paprika, garlic powder and pepper and rub all other them. Remember to turn them over and coat all sides with this seasoning. Now wrap in the aluminum foil, but leave one end open, as into this you will then pour the water. Now fold up the open end to seal the meat inside. It is a good idea to leave some room around the meat to allow heat inside to then circulate when the ribs are cooking.

2. When it comes to cooking these on the barbecue you place them on the grill and pull the lid down and leave them there for between 45 minutes and an hour. Once the time has elapsed remove the ribs from the tin foil and then replace them on the grill, which has been lightly oiled.

3. After placing the ribs on the grill you can now start basting them with the barbecue sauce. You should allow them to remain on the grill for a further 10 to 15 minutes. During this final cooking time you should be turning them over every 5 minutes and brushing them with the sauce each time they are turned.

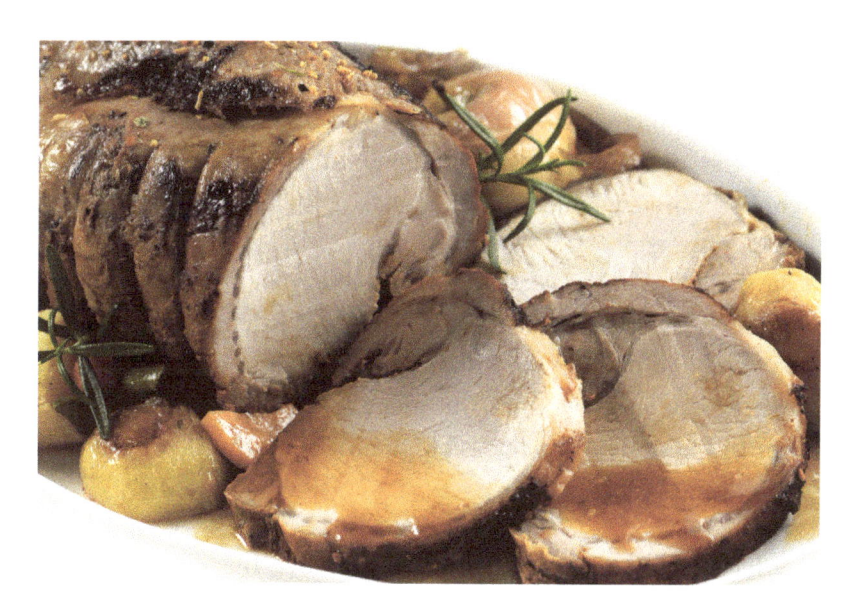

RECIPE 11 – MAPLE GARLIC PORK TENDERLOIN

The adding of garlic to the marinade helps to counteract some of the maple sweetness.

Barbecue Cookbook

Ingredients

680gram Pork Tenderloin

2 Tablespoons Dijon Mustard

1 Teaspoon Sesame Oil

3 Garlic Cloves Minced

240ml Maple Syrup

Freshly Ground Black Pepper

Instructions

1. In a bowl mix together the maple syrup, mustard, sesame oil, garlic and pepper. Whisk thoroughly to ensure that all these ingredients are combined together well.

2. In a shallow dish place the pork tenderloin and then coat it thoroughly with the marinade that you have just made. Cover the meat over and place in the refrigerator to chill for at least 8 hours. However if you really want the meat to absorb as much of the flavor of the marinade as possible then it is best to leave it in the refrigerator overnight.

3. Whilst the barbecue is heating up remove the pork from the refrigerator so that it can come up to room temperature. Once the barbecue is hot enough remove the meat from the dish and set over to one side. As for any sauce left in the dish pour this into a small saucepan.

4. Now before you place the meat on the grill make sure you have brushed it with some oil first to prevent the meat from sticking to it. Cook the pork on the particular for between 15 and 25 minutes

making sure that you baste it regularly with the reserved marinade, which you have heated up in the saucepan for five minutes first. Make sure that you cook the meat on a medium heat otherwise the marinade will burn. Plus of course remember to turn the meat regularly to ensure that it is cooked through evenly.

As soon as the meat is cooked the inside no longer looks pink place to one side for a few minutes before carving and serving to your guests.

RECIPE 12 – MAPLE GLAZED RIBS

The sweetness of the maple syrup really does help to bring out the lovely taste of this meat.

Ingredients

1.5kg Baby Back Pork Ribs

180ml Maple Syrup

2 Tablespoons Brown Sugar

2 Tablespoons Ketchup

1 Tablespoon Cider Vinegar

1 Tablespoon Worcestershire Sauce

½ Teaspoon Salt

½ Teaspoon Mustard Powder

Instructions

1. Place the ribs into a large saucepan or pot and cover with water. Then cook on a low heat so the water is simmering for at least an hour or until the meat has become tender. Once the meat is cooked remove the ribs from the water and place them in a shallow dish and set aside whilst you make the marinade.

2. To make the marinade place the maple syrup, sugar, ketchup, vinegar, Worcestershire sauce, salt and mustard into a saucepan. Place on the hob and bring to the ingredients to the boil before then reducing the heat down and cooking for five minutes. Make sure that you stir the sauce frequently then allow to cool slightly before then pouring it over the ribs. Now place the ribs in the dish covered in the sauce in the refrigerator for 2 hours to marinate.

3. You will be cooking the ribs on an indirect heat on the grill so make sure that it is hot enough. Once the barbecue has heated up sufficiently remove the ribs from the marinade and place them on the lightly oiled barbecue grill. Any marinade left over should be put into a saucepan and boiled for a few minutes.

4. The ribs should only need to remain on the barbecue for around 20 minutes. During this time they should be turned frequently and brushed with the cooked marinade often until the ribs have become nicely glazed. Divide up the ribs into manageable portions and serve to your guests.

RECIPE 13 – SMOKED PORK SPARE RIBS

These are slightly sweet but also slightly spicy yet the flavors don't overwhelm the meat, which falls away from the bone very easily when cooked properly.

Samantha Michaels

Ingredients

3Kg Pork Spareribs

Dry Rub Mixture

64gram Brown Sugar

2 Tablespoons Chili Powder

1 Tablespoon Paprika

1 Tablespoon Freshly Ground Black Pepper

2 Tablespoons Garlic Powder

2 Teaspoons Onion Powder

2 Teaspoons Salt

2 Teaspoons Ground Cumin

1 Teaspoon Ground Cinnamon

1 Teaspoon Cayenne Pepper

1 Teaspoon Jalapeno Seasoning Salt (Optional)

Sauce

240ml Apple Cider

180ml Apple Cider Vinegar

Barbecue Cookbook

1 Tablespoon Onion Powder

1 Tablespoon Garlic Powder

2 Tablespoons Fresh Lemon Juice

1 Finely Chopped Jalapeno Pepper (Optional)

3 Tablespoons Hot Pepper Sauce

Salt

Freshly Ground Black Pepper

2 Cups Of Soaked Wood Chips

Instructions

1. In a bowl place the brown sugar, chili powder, paprika, black pepper, garlic powder, onion powder, salt, cumin, cinnamon, jalapeno seasoning and cayenne pepper and mix well together. Then rub all over the spareribs, cover and put in the refrigerator for at least 4 hours to allow the rub to become infused in to the meat. However leaving them overnight would prove even better.

2. Whilst the barbecue is heating up you should now remove the spareribs from the refrigerator and start preparing the sauce. In a bowl you need to place all the ingredients mentioned above and stir together.

3. Once the barbecue is ready before you place the spareribs on the lightly oiled grill you must first place some of the soaked wood chips on to the barbecue itself. Once you have done this you can now place the spareribs on the grill with the bone at the bottom. Now close the lid and allow the ribs to cook for between 3 ½ to 4 hours. If you need to add more coals then do so.

4. Every hour you will need to baste the ribs with the sauce and also make sure at this time you also add some more of the soaked wood chips to the barbecue. It is important that the temperature within the remains at a constant 225 degrees Fahrenheit to ensure that the pork spareribs cook properly.

You can tell when the ribs are ready to eat as the rub will have help to create a crispy blackened bark on the meat and it pulls away from the bone easily. Simply separate into portions that your guests can enjoy and discard any sauce that may be left over.

RECIPE 14 – BOURBON PORK RIBS

Even though you can cook these ribs in the oven it really is best if you cook them on the barbecue, as this helps to enhance the flavor of the marinade further. Once cooked serve them with a delicious crispy green salad and some garlic cheese potatoes.

Ingredients

1.36Kg Pork Ribs (Country Style Ones If You Can Get Them)

128gram Dark Brown Sugar

240ml Light Soy Sauce

150ml Bourbon

4 Garlic Cloves Minced

Instructions

1. In a food processor or blender place the sugar, soy sauce, garlic and bourbon and turn on until all ingredients are thoroughly combined. Now pour this mixture over the ribs, which have been placed in a shallow dish.

2. Cover the ribs and place them in a refrigerator to marinate for several hours. The longer you leave them in the refrigerator then the more the marinate will infuse into the rib meat.

3. Whilst the barbecue is heating up you should remove the ribs from the refrigerator to allow them to come up to room temperature. But before you place them on the barbecue grate make sure it has been brushed with oil.

4. Once the ribs are on the grate you now need to close the lid and cook them for between 45 minutes and an hour. How long you cook them for will depend on how thick the ribs are. The best way to test if they are ready to eat is to insert a meat thermometer into the thickest part of the rib. If the internal temperature measures 160 degrees Fahrenheit they are ready to serve up on to plates after being separated with the salad and potatoes.

RECIPE 15 - MARGARITA GLAZED PORK CHOPS

This really is a recipe that will excite your taste buds as well as provide you with a food that really does bring out the summer in you.

Ingredients

4 Boneless Pork Loin Chops That Are About 1 Inch Thick

160ml Orange Marmalade

1 Jalapeno Pepper Seeded And Finely Chopped

2 Tablespoons Lime Juice or Tequila

1 Teaspoon Freshly Grated Ginger (If you don't have fresh ginger use ½ teaspoon ground ginger instead)

Instructions

1. In a bowl mix together the marmalade, jalapeno pepper, lime juice or tequila and the ginger. This is what will be used to glaze the pork chops.

2. Before you place the chops on the grill making sure that they cook over a medium heat you trim off the fat.

3. Allow the chops to cook on the barbecue for between 12 and 15 minutes dependent on the thickness of them. The best way of testing to see if they are ready to eat is to insert a skewer into the thickest part and see if the juices from inside that come out run clear. It is also important that you turn the chops over regularly when cooking them.

4. During the last five minutes of the chops cooking this is when the glaze you made earlier must be applied. During this time the chops should only be turned once, but you must apply the glaze often.

5. Once the chops are ready to eat remove from the barbecue and place on clean plates then sprinkle with a little chopped fresh cilantro and some orange and lime wedges.

Chapter 4 - Lamb Recipes

Recipe 1 – Lamb Chops With Curry, Apple And Raisin Sauce

The curry, apple and raisin sauce that you use with this particular recipe helps to enhance the flavor of the lamb further. Plus adds a little bit of spice to the recipe as well.

Ingredients

6 Lamb Chops (Each weighing around 115gram)

1 Teaspoon Salt to season meat

Sauce

57gram Butter

1 Tablespoon Olive Oil

384gram Chopped Onion

1 Crushed Garlic Clove

2 Tablespoons Curry Powder

1 Tablespoon Ground Coriander

1 Tablespoon Ground Cumin

2 Teaspoons Salt To Season

Samantha Michaels

2 Teaspoons White Pepper To Season

1 Teaspoon Dried Thyme

½ Lemon Seeded and Finely Chopped (Peel As Well)

384gram Apples Peeled, Cored and Chopped

128gram Apple Sauce

85gram Dark Raisins

85gram Golden Raisins

1 Tablespoon Water (If Needed)

Instructions

1. In a saucepan place the butter, olive oil, onions and garlic and cook them over a medium heat until the onions have turned translucent. This should take around 8 minutes to happen. Once the onions are ready you stir in the rest of the ingredients to make the sauce and bring the mixture to the boil.

As soon as the mixture has started to boil you now need to turn the heat down and cover the saucepan and let the mixture simmer for a while. You should check the sauce regularly and stir it also to make sure that it doesn't stick to the saucepan. You will know when it is ready because it will have the consistency of apple sauce and the raisins will start to break apart. Expect this part of the process to take an hour to happen. However if you notice the mixture is becoming thick then stir in the tablespoon of water.

2. Once the sauce is ready you can now go ahead and cook the lamb chops. However before you place on the grill make sure that it has been lightly oiled and that the chops have been seasoned

with some salt. Leave them on the grill until the outside has started to turn a golden brown, which should be around 3 to 5 minutes for each side. Of course how long you cook them for will depend on whether you want the meat to be medium rare or medium inside.

To further help test if they are ready insert a meat thermometer into the chop making sure it isn't touching the bone and the internal temperature should have reached 145 degrees Fahrenheit. When the lamb chops are cooked place on clean plates and in a small bowl beside them place the sauce made earlier.

Recipe 2 – Grilled Lamb With Brown Sugar Glaze

Looking for something quick and easy to prepare at a barbecue this summer then this recipe should be tried.

Ingredients

4 Lamb Chops

32gram Brown Sugar

2 Teaspoons Ground Ginger

2 Teaspoons Dried Tarragon

1 Teaspoon Ground Cinnamon

1 Teaspoon Ground Black Pepper

1 Teaspoon Garlic Powder

½ Teaspoon Salt

Samantha Michaels

Instructions

1. In a bowl place the sugar, ginger, cinnamon, tarragon, pepper, garlic powder and salt and mix well together.

2. Now take this seasoning mixture and rub well into the lamb chops on both sides then place on a place and cover. Then place in the refrigerator for an hour.

3. To cook the lamb chops you must remove them from the refrigerator whilst the barbecue is heating up to bring them back up to room temperature and they need to be cooked on a high heat.

4. As usual brush the grill of the barbecue with some oil first before laying the chops on it. Then cook the chops on each side for around 5 minutes or until they are cooked the way you like them. Once they are cooked allow them to rest for a few minutes before serving with a salad and some new potatoes.

RECIPE 3 – MEDITERRANEAN LAMB BURGERS

These burgers really do help to make a barbecue feel even more special. You should serve the burgers in buns with a little salad and feta cheese and also a yoghurt dip.

Ingredients

Burgers

450gram Ground Lamb

225gram Ground Beef

3 Tablespoons Freshly Chopped Mint

1 Teaspoon Freshly Minced Ginger Root

1 Teaspoon Minced Garlic

1 Teaspoon Salt

½ Teaspoon Freshly Ground Black Pepper

Yogurt Sauce

450gram Greek Yogurt

Zest Of ½ Lemon

1 Minced Garlic Clove

½ Teaspoon Salt

Instructions

1. To make the burgers you place the ground lamb and beef in to a bowl with the mint, ginger root, garlic, salt and pepper and stir together until just about combined. Now divide the mixture up into four portions then shape them into four patties. Set them aside. It is best if you cover them up and place in the refrigerator until you are ready to cook them.

2. After making the burgers you are now ready to make the sauce. To do this place the yogurt, lemon zest, garlic and salt into a bowl and mix well. Place the mixture, which you have covered over, into the refrigerator until it is needed.

3. When it comes to cooking the lamb the barbecue should be at a medium heat and will need to be cooked on both sides for between 3 and 4 minutes each. The best way to test to see if they are cooked through is to insert a meat thermometer and see if the temperature inside them has reached 160 degrees Fahrenheit.

4. Once the burgers are ready you need to prepare the buns in which the burgers will be served. The first thing you should do is place a slice of onion and tomato on the grill and cook them until they are lightly charred on each side. Then spread some of the yogurt sauce over the burger or ciabatta roll and then place the burger on top of this. Then place on top of this the onion and tomato slices before some leaves of lettuce. Then top it all off with some slices of feta cheese and the top part of the roll.

RECIPE 4 – GRILLED LAMB CHOPS

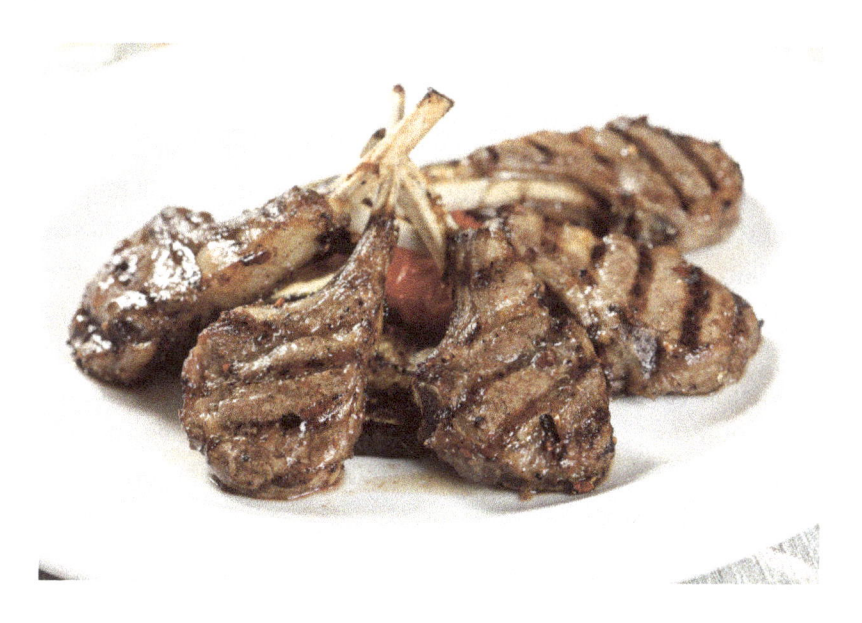

Looking for a recipe that will not need much time dedicated to preparing it but will still taste absolutely wonderful after being cooked on the barbecue then you should try this recipe out.

Barbecue Cookbook

Ingredients

900gram Lamb Chops

60ml Distilled White Vinegar

2 Teaspoons Salt

½ Teaspoon Ground Black Pepper

1 Tablespoon Minced Garlic

1 Thinly Sliced Onion

2 Tablespoons Olive Oil

Instructions

1. In a large resealable bag place the vinegar, salt, pepper, garlic, onion and olive oil and shake well to ensure that all the ingredients have been combined together properly. Then into the bag you place the chops again shake the bag vigorously as this will help to ensure that the chops have been thoroughly coated with the marinate. Once this has been done you place the bag into the refrigerator and leave there for 2 hours.

2. When it comes to cooking the lamb chops you should remove them from the refrigerator whilst the barbecue is heating up. This will ensure that they come up to room temperature ensuring that they then cook properly.

3. When you remove the lamb chops from the marinade to place on the lightly oiled grill if you notice any pieces of onion stuck to them leave them in place. Then grill them until they are cooked to the level of doneness you require. Around 3 minutes for each side

should be enough for them to be medium. Once cooked allow to rest for a short while before then serving to your guests.

RECIPE 5 – LAMB KOFTA KEBABS

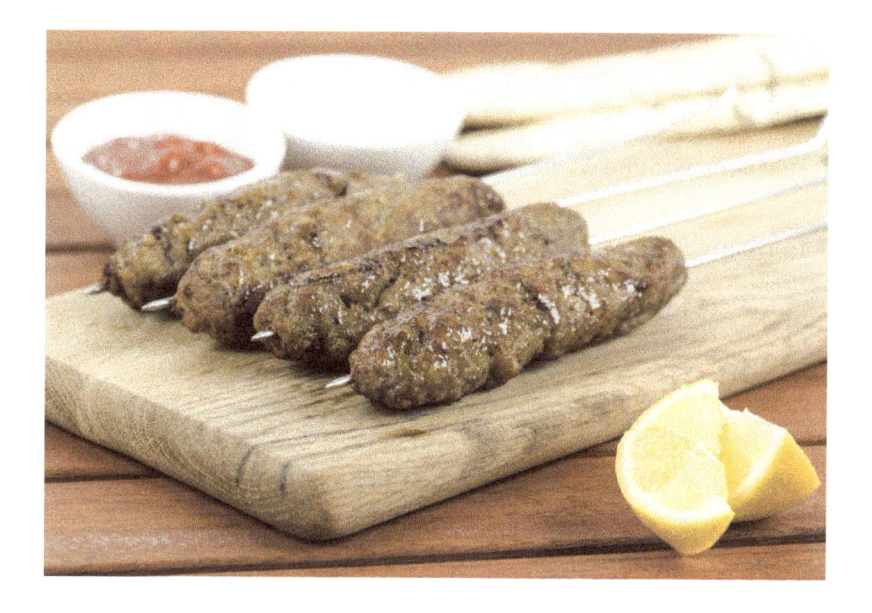

These lamb Kofta kebabs don't take very long to prepare or cook and make a wonderful addition to any barbecue.

Ingredients

450gram Ground Lamb Meat

4 Garlic Cloves Minced

1 Teaspoon Salt

3 Tablespoons Grated Onion

3 Tablespoons Freshly Chopped Parsley

1 Tablespoon Ground Coriander

1 Teaspoon Ground Cumin

½ Teaspoon Ground Cinnamon

½ Teaspoon Ground All Spice

¼ Teaspoon Cayenne Pepper

¼ Teaspoon Ground Ginger

¼ Teaspoon Freshly Ground Black Pepper

Instructions

1. With a mortar and pestle ground the garlic into a paste with the salt then the place these ingredients into a bowl with the onion, parsley, coriander, cumin, cinnamon, all spice, cayenne pepper, ginger and black pepper then to this bowl add the ground lamb meat.

2. Once all the above ingredients have been combined together divide it in to 28 small pieces and form them into balls.

3. To make the Kofta kebabs take one of the balls of meat and thread it on to the top of a wooden skewer that has been soaking in water for ½ hour. Then very slowly start to flatten the meat down the skewer until a 2 inch oval is created. Do this with all 28 balls of meat and then place them on a clean plate, cover and put in to the refrigerator for between 30 minutes and 12 hours.

4. To cook the Lamb Kofta Kebabs you need to ensure that the temperature of the barbecue is of a medium heat and the grill has been lightly oiled. Once the barbecue has reached the right

temperature place the kebabs on the grill and cook for around 6 minutes, making sure that you turn them over regularly.

Recipe 6 – Barbecued Asian Butterflied Leg Of Lamb

As this recipe does take quite a bit of time to prepare this is the kind of meal you should be serving at a barbecue for a special occasion such as a wedding anniversary celebration.

Ingredients

2.26Kg Boneless Butterflied Leg Of Lamb (Ask your butcher to prepare the meat for you)

75ml Hoisin Sauce

6 Tablespoons Rice Vinegar

64gram Minced Green Onions

50ml Mushroom Soy Sauce

4 Tablespoons Minced Garlic

2 Tablespoons Honey

½ Teaspoon Sesame Oil

1 Tablespoon Toasted Sesame Seeds

½ Teaspoon Freshly Ground White Pepper

½ Teaspoon Freshly Ground Black Pepper

Barbecue Cookbook

Instructions

1. Place the hoisin sauce, rice vinegar, green onions, mushroom soy sauce, honey, garlic, sesame oil, sesame seeds, white and black pepper into a resealable plastic bag and shake vigorously as this will help to ensure that all the ingredients are mixed together properly.

2. Once you have made the marinade now place the leg of lamb into the bag also and seal it and move the bag around to ensure that all the meat is coated in the marinade. After doing this you should place the bag in the refrigerator for at least 8 hours. But it is best to leave it in the bag in the refrigerator overnight.

3. Whilst the barbecue is heating up you should now remove the meat from the refrigerator and leave it in the bag until the barbecue is hot enough to cook the meat on it.

4. Before placing the meat on the grill brush some oil over its surface and then place the lamb on top. Any marinade left over should be discarded.

5. You should be looking to cook each side for of the meat for around 15 minutes or until you feel it done to the way you enjoy eating lamb. If you are unsure if the lamb is ready and you have a meat thermometer then insert this to check the internal temperature. The meat should be ready when the internal temperature has reached 145 degrees Fahrenheit.

6. As soon as the lamb is cooked remove from the heat and place on a clean plate and allow it to rest for 20 minutes, remembering to keep it covered whilst resting. Then slice and serve.

Recipe 7 – Summer Lamb Kebabs

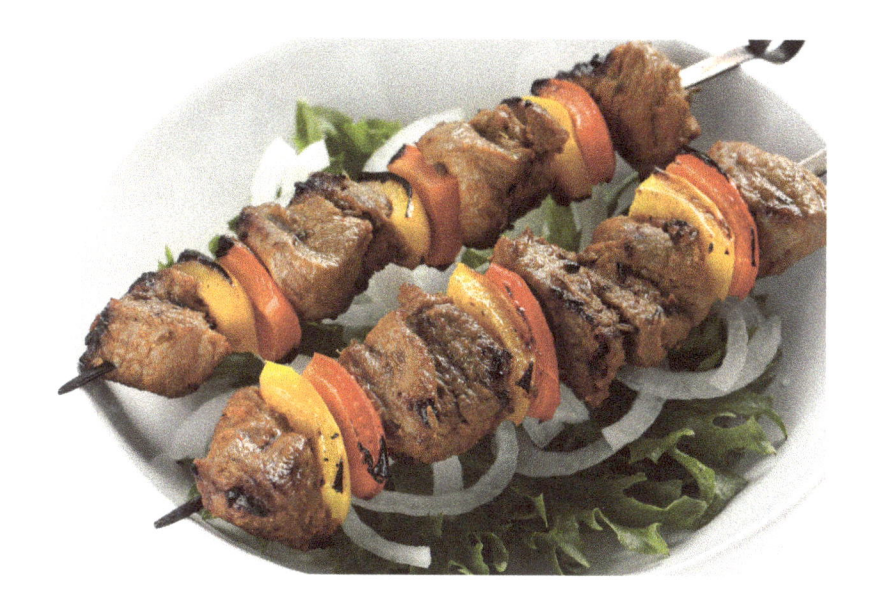

A very unusual recipe but one that really helps to enhance the beautiful flavors of the lamb.

Ingredients

2.26Kg Boneless Lamb Shoulder Cut Into 1 Inch Chunks

6 Tablespoons Dijon Mustard

4 Tablespoons White Wine Vinegar

4 Tablespoons Olive Oil

½ Teaspoon Salt

½ Teaspoon Freshly Ground Black Pepper

½ Teaspoon Freshly Chopped Rosemary

Barbecue Cookbook

½ Teaspoon Dried Crumbled Sage

4 Garlic Cloves Chopped

4 Green Bell Peppers Cut Into Large Chunks

1 Packet Fresh Whole Mushrooms (The Button Type Are Ideal)

1 Can Pineapple Chunks (Juice Drained But Retained)

256gram Cherry Tomatoes

4 Onions Cut Into Quarters

1 Jar Maraschino Cherries (Juice Drained But Retained)

76gram Butter Or Margarine Melted

Instructions

1. In a large bowl put the chunks of lamb ready for the marinade to be added to them.

2. To make the marinade place the mustard, vinegar, olive oil, salt, pepper, sage, rosemary and garlic and mix well together before then pouring over the lamb. Use your hands and mix all these ingredients together to make sure that all parts of the lamb are then coated in the marinade. Once you have done this cover the bowl over and place in the refrigerator overnight.

3. Whilst the barbecue is heating up you can now start to make the kebabs. If you are using wooden skewers make sure that they have been soaking in some water for at least 30 minutes. To make each kebab thread on pieces of meat along with some of the mushrooms, tomatoes, pineapple and cherries and then place on the lightly oiled barbecue grill to cook. Each kebab should remain

on the barbecue for around 12 minutes and you should be turning them over frequently to prevent them from burning.

4. It is important that whilst cooking the kebabs that you baste them with a sauce made from the melted butter, pineapple and cherry juice. This will help to enhance the flavor not only of the lamb but the other ingredients on the kebabs.

RECIPE 8 – HERB MARINATED LAMB CHOPS

Although this recipe requires the lamb chops to remain in the marinade for 8 hours or more it helps to make the meat much more tender. Plus helps the marinade being absorbed by the meat and so helps to bring out more of its flavor.

Ingredients

4 Lamb Loin Chops Bone In (1 Inch Thick)

60ml Dry Red Wine

2 Tablespoons Sodium Reduced Soy Sauce

1 ½ Teaspoons Fresh Minced Basil

½ Teaspoon Freshly Ground Pepper

1 Minced Garlic Clove

Instructions

1. In a large plastic resealable bag mix together the wine, soy sauce, basil, mint, garlic and pepper. Once thoroughly mixed together pop the chops into the bag and shake the bag so that all

Barbecue Cookbook

parts of the chops are coated in the refrigerator. Now seal the back up and place in the refrigerator for at least 8 hours. However if you have enough time available leave them in the refrigerator overnight.

2. Whilst the barbecue is heating up remove the lamb chops from the refrigerator and from the bag. Any marinade left in the bag should be discarded.

3. Once the barbecue is at the right temperature you need to be cooking the lamb chops over a medium heat with the cover up. To cook the chops on a medium heat the grill, which has been lightly oiled, should sit about 4 to 6 inches above the heat source. Now cook each side of the chop for between 5 and 7 minutes or until the meat has reached the way you like lamb to be cooked.

When the lamb chops are cooked remove from heat and let them rest for a short while before serving. A good accompaniment to serve with this particular recipe would be some couscous.

RECIPE 9 – GRILLED INDIAN STYLE LAMB CHOPS

These particular lamb chops after being removed from the marinade will need to be cooked hot and fast. A good accompaniment to serve with this particular dish would be some rice or some grilled vegetables.

Ingredients

12 Lamb Rib Chops

60ml Water

3 Tablespoons Vegetable Oil

2 Tablespoons Curry Powder

1 Tablespoon White Vinegar

2 Teaspoons Onion Powder

1 Teaspoon Garlic Powder

1 Teaspoon Garam Masala

¼ Teaspoon Salt

Instructions

1. Place the 12 lamb rib chops into a shallow dish. Now in a bowl mix together the oil, curry powder, white vinegar, onion and garlic powder, the garam masala and salt and then pour this over the lamb chops. It is a good to pour ½ the marinade over first then turn the chops over and pour the rest of the marinade over them.

2. You now need to place the dish, which you have covered over, in the refrigerator for 1 to 3 hours. Remove them from the refrigerator at least 15 minutes before required in order to bring the meat back up to room temperature.

3. Whilst waiting for the chops to comeback up to room temperature now is when you should light the barbecue so it will be hot enough for you to then cook the lamb rib chops on it very quickly. In fact you need to cook the lamb chops on the barbecue on a medium heat so the grill should sit around 4 to 6 inches above the heat source.

4. When it comes to cooking the lamb chops they should be cooked on each side for 4 minutes. However before you place them on the grill make sure that you have oiled it well. Once the chops are

cooked they can be served immediately with either some chutney or a yogurt sauce.

RECIPE 10 – MOROCCAN LEG OF LAMB

Not only is this an exotic way to serve a leg of lamb to your guests but also a very flavorsome way.

Ingredients

1.36 to 1.81Kg Boneless Leg of Lamb

43gram Freshly Chopped Cilantro

32gram Freshly Chopped Mint

60ml Olive Oil

2 Minced Garlic Cloves

2 Teaspoons Ground Coriander

1 Teaspoon Freshly Grated Ginger

1 Teaspoon Salt

½ Teaspoon Chili Powder

Instructions

1. In a small mix together the oil, cilantro, mint, garlic, coriander, ginger, salt and chilli powder.

2. Place the boneless leg of lamb into a shallow dish and then pour over the marinade you have just made. Cover the dish with some aluminum foil and place in the refrigerator for it to then marinate for between 2 and 4 hours.

3. When the time comes to remove the lamb from the refrigerator you should now start heating up the barbecue. Make sure that it is heated up to a temperature that allows you to cook the lamb on a medium to low heat.

4. As soon as the barbecue is ready place the leg of lamb on to the grill, which has been oiled before, and cook directly above the heat source for 20 to 30 minutes or until it has cooked to the way you like it. Once the lamb has cooked remove from the barbecue and place on a clean plate to rest for 10 minutes before you then carve and serve it. A nice accompaniment to this particular dish would be a fresh green bean salad and some couscous or rice.

Recipe 11 – South African Lamb And Apricot Sosaties (Kebabs)

This is a very traditional style of South African barbecue (braai) dish and if you want you can replace the lamb with beef or venison.

Ingredients

200gram Diced Lamb

225gram Low Fat Natural Yogurt

350gram Dried Apricots

1 Dessertspoon Curry Powder

Barbecue Cookbook

1 Tablespoon Caster Sugar

1 Tablespoon Vegetable Oil

1 Large Onion

Instructions

1. In a bowl combine together the yogurt; curry powder, sugar and oil to make a sauce. Add as much salt and pepper to this to season.

2. Take the onion and cut this in 1 ¼ inch pieces which you will then thread on to the skewers alternately with the diced lamb and the dried apricots. If you are going to be using wooden skewers then make sure that you soak them in some water for around 30 minutes before you make the Sosaties.

3. Once you have threaded all the lamb, apricot and onions on to the skewers place them in a large plastic resealable bag or a container then pour the sauce you made previously all over them. If you need to do turn the kebabs over to ensure that they are well coated with the sauce that you are now going to marinate them in. You can either leave them to marinate in the sauce for 8 hours. However if you want the Sosaties to become infused with lots of the marinate's flavor it is best to leave them in it in a refrigerator overnight.

4. When it comes to cooking the Sosaties preheat the barbecue to a medium heat and just before you lay the Sosaties on the grill brush it with some oil. Cook the Sosaties on the grill for 8 to 10 minutes on each side. Then remove from the heat and serve immediately to your guests.

Recipe 12 – Greek Lamb Chops

Not only are these lamb chops packed with loads of flavor if you leave them in the marinade for some time they come out tasting extremely tender.

Ingredients

8 Lamb Chops

120ml Olive Oil

120ml Red Wine Vinegar

32gram Freshly Chopped Mint

3 Cloves Garlic Minced

1 Teaspoon Salt

1 Teaspoon Freshly Ground Black Pepper

Instructions

1. In a bowl combine together the olive oil, red wine vinegar, freshly chopped mint and minced garlic cloves. Now pour this mixture (marinade) into a bag that is resealable and to this add the lamb chops. Move the chops around inside the bag to ensure that they are well coated in the marinade and place in the refrigerator. Leave them there for 2 hours.

2. After removing the lamb chops from the refrigerator you should pre heat the barbecue in readiness for when they will need cooking.

3. Before placing the lamb chops on the grill you should season with a little salt and pepper. Then after making sure that the grill of the barbecue is about 3 inches above the heat source you should oil it lightly before placing the chops on it.

4. You should cook each chop for 5 to 6 minutes on each side. It is a good idea to turn them over regularly to prevent them from burning rather than just charring. Once the cooking time has elapsed remove from heat and place on a clean plate to rest for a few minutes. Then serve them with some pitta bread, yogurt dip and a Greek salad.

RECIPE 13 – GRILLED RACK OF LAMB

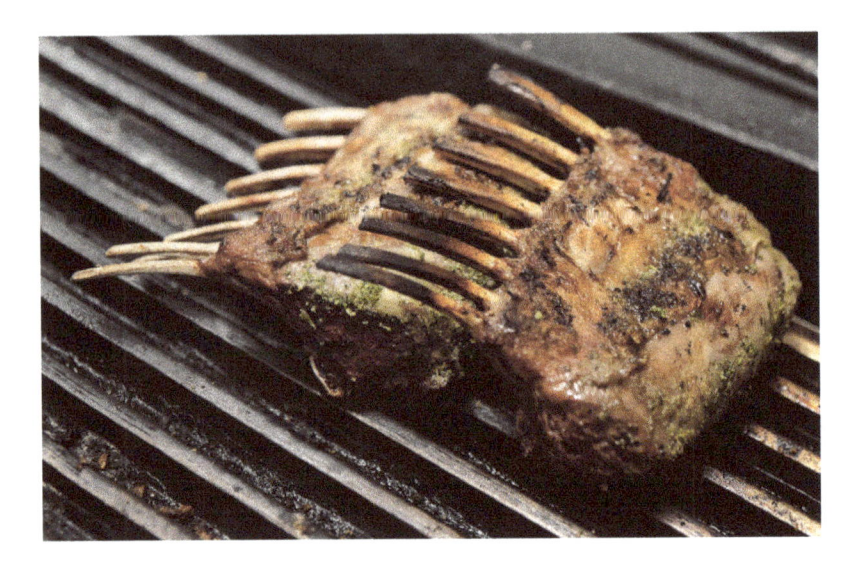

The marinade you make for this particular dish helps to give the lamb a much sweeter and tarter flavor helping to enhance the meat even more.

Samantha Michaels

Ingredients

1 Rack Of Lamb

240ml Red Currant Jelly

240ml Dijon Mustard

240ml White Wine (Dry or Medium Would Be Best)

64gram Butter

64gram Minced Shallots

2 Tablespoons Fresh Crushed Rosemary

Instructions

1. In a saucepan place the red currant jelly and mustard and simmer on a low heat for about 5 minutes or until the jelly has melted. Then allow the sauce to cool completely.

2. Cut the rack of lamb into chops and then French cut. If you are not able to do this then get your butcher to do it for you. It is important if you decide to do this yourself that you don't remove any of the fat from the eye of the chop. This fat actually helps to prevent the meat from burning when you place it on the barbecue grill.

3. Once the rack of lamb is ready you now submerge it completely in the sauce you made earlier and leave it in it to marinade overnight. Cover the dish in which the lamb has been placed and put in the refrigerator.

4. When it comes to cooking the lamb it should be done over a medium to high heat and with some hickory coals added to the

barbecue beforehand. Also make sure that the grill has been oiled before the lamb is placed on it. Cook on the barbecue for 4 to 5 minutes on each side and basting each side regularly with more of the marinade sauce.

5. Whilst the lamb is resting you can now prepare the garnish to go with them. In a saucepan place the butter and allow it to melt over a low heat then add the minced shallots to it. Allow the shallots to brown before then adding the crushed rosemary and white wine.

As soon as the garnish is ready place the lamb on clean plates and serve with the garnish poured over it and with grilled vegetables and potatoes.

RECIPE 14 – GREEK BURGERS

To further add a real Greek feel to these burgers it is a good idea to add some feta cheese to the top of burgher just before serving.

Ingredients

450gram Ground Lamb

1 Tablespoon Dijon Mustard

1 Tablespoon Fresh Lemon Juice

1 Tablespoon Minced Onion

1 Garlic Clove Minced

½ Teaspoon Crushed Dried Rosemary

½ Teaspoon Salt (To Taste)

¼ Teaspoon Freshly Ground Pepper

To Serve

4 Hamburger Rolls or Pitta Breads

Cucumber Slices

Tomato Slices

Onion Slices

Instructions

1. In a bowl mix together the ground lamb, mustard, lemon juice, onion, garlic, rosemary, salt and pepper. You can of course combine these ingredients by hand otherwise you may want to consider using a food processor.

2. Once all the above ingredients have been combined together you now need to divide into four equal portions and then form patties out of each one. It is important that whilst you are making these Greek burgers that you turn the barbecue on or light the coals so it is at the right temperature for you to then cook the burgers.

3. Before you place the burgers on the grill lightly oil its surface with some olive oil and grill until you notice the burgers are no longer pink in color. On average you should expect it to take around 10 minutes for these burgers to be cooked properly. Remember to turn them over at least once.

4. Just before you take the burgers off the grill place the pitta breads or burger buns on it to become warmed through. Then when they are ready place the burgers on them and top with slices

of cucumber, tomato and onion. You may also want to consider adding a light yogurt and mint dressing to them as well.

Recipe 15 – Teriyaki Lamb Kebabs

Most people wouldn't consider using teriyaki sauce on lamb but it does actually compliment the meat very well. These lamb kebabs make a wonderful meal for a warm summer evening when served with some rice.

Ingredients

680gram Boneless Lamb Cut Into 1 Inch Cubes

3 Bell Peppers (1 Red, 1 Yellow and 1 Green) Deseeded And Cut Into 1 Inch Pieces

2 Medium Red Onions Cut Into 1 Inch Pieces

8 Cap Mushrooms

1 Pineapple Cut Into 1 Inch Pieces

Marinade

60ml Red Wine

2 Tablespoons Olive Oil

2 Tablespoons Teriyaki Sauce

4 Cloves of Garlic Minced

Grated Rind Of 1 Lemon

1 Teaspoon Freshly Ground Black Pepper

½ Teaspoon Ground Ginger (Fresh If Possible)

Instructions

1. In a bowl mix together all the marinade ingredients then place to one side.

2. Now on to skewers thread pieces of the lamb, peppers, onions, mushrooms and pineapple. Alternate between each item and if you are using wooden skewers then make sure that they have been soaked in some water for at least 30 minutes before you start making the kebabs.

3. As you make each kebab place them in a shallow dish and when all have been made you can now pour over the marinade. Pour over the marinade a little at the time and turn the kebabs over to ensure that every part of them is coated in the marinade. Now cover and place in the refrigerator for at least 8 hours. Whilst they are in the refrigerator make sure that you turn them over occasionally to ensure that all sides of the kebabs remain coated in the marinade.

4. After removing the lamb kebabs from the refrigerator you should start your barbecue up this will then allow time for the kebabs to reach room temperature and will help to make cooking them much easier. You should cook them over a medium heat so place the grill about 6 inches above the heat source.

5. Prior to placing the kebabs on the grill apply a little olive to prevent the kebabs from sticking to it. Then brush with some of the left over marinade and cook for between 12 and 15 minutes.

Barbecue Cookbook

Whilst they are cooking make sure that you turn them over at least 3 times to ensure that they cooked evenly through. Once they are cooked serve immediately to your guests.

Chapter 5 - Fish Recipes

Recipe 1 – Fresh Citrus Salmon

This particular recipe comes with quite a tangy taste, which helps to enhance the flavor of the salmon further.

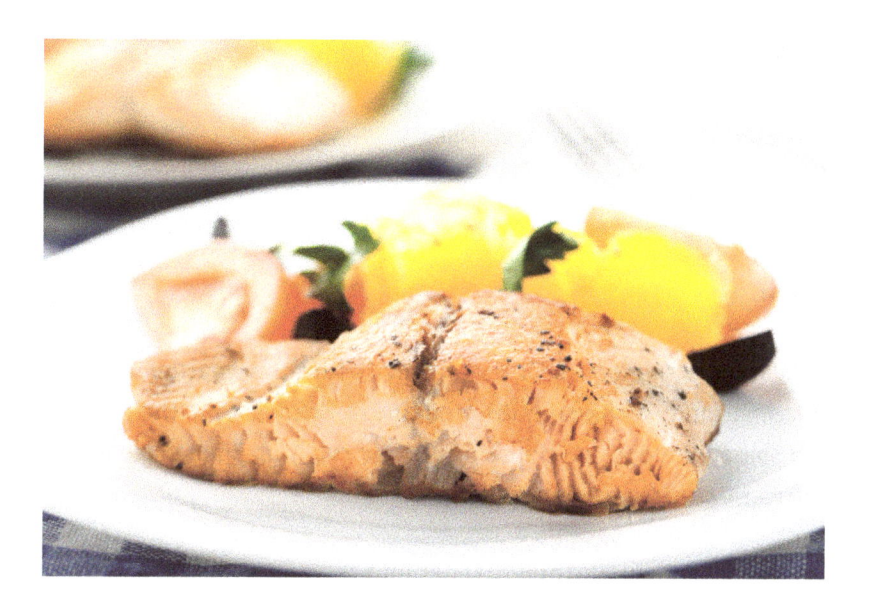

Ingredients

4 Salmon Fillets With Skin Left On

2 Small Lemons

2 Medium Oranges

1 Large Lime

100ml Freshly Squeezed Lemon Juice

100ml Freshly Squeezed Orange Juice

2 Large Garlic Cloves Divided

Freshly Ground Black Pepper

Sea Salt

50ml Freshly Squeezed Lime Juice

Olive Oil

4 Tablespoons Balsamic Vinegar

2 Teaspoons Freshly Chopped Dill

Instructions

1. Wash the salmon fillets thoroughly before then patting dry and drizzling them with some olive oil and sprinkling over them some sea salt and pepper on the skin side and rub it in. Then place in the refrigerator for 30 minutes.

2. Cut the lemon, lime and oranges into segments making sure that you retain as much of their juices as possible. Then mix these segments with some olive oil and ½ crushed garlic clove. Now place in the refrigerator.

3. Next you need to combine the freshly cut dill with 1 garlic clove that has been crushed, the lime, lemon and orange juice and a little olive oil, salt and pepper. Once you have done this you remove the salmon fillets from the refrigerator and place them in a shallow dish and pour over this marinade. Cover the dish and replace in the refrigerator and leave the salmon to marinate in the dill for at least 2 hours.

4. Once two hours is up remove the salmon fillets from the refrigerator and as the barbecue warms up this will allow them to

come up to room temperature. Allow the salmon to be out of the refrigerator for 20 minutes before you then place on the barbecue.

5. Before you place the salmon on the barbecue rub the grate with a clove of garlic and then place the fish on it skin side down. After two minutes you must turn the salmon over and allow it to cook for a further two minutes. Also it is important to place some sort of cover over the salmon such as saucepan lid that is well ventilated. Once cooked let the salmon fillets rest for 3 minutes before serving. When you serve the salmon place on the plate a small salad made up of lettuce, cherry tomatoes and drizzle some balsamic vinegar around the plate.

RECIPE 2 – MARINATED BARBECUED SWORDFISH

The use of white wine, soy sauce, garlic and lemon juice help to bring out more of the swordfishes amazing flavor as well as help to cook it better on the barbecue.

Ingredients

4 Swordfish Steaks

4 Garlic Cloves

75ml White Wine

4 Tablespoons Lemon Juice

2 Tablespoons Soy Sauce

2 Tablespoons Olive Oil

1 Tablespoon Savory Seasoning

¼ Teaspoon Salt

1/8 Teaspoon Freshly Ground Black Pepper

Instructions

1. In a shallow dish you whisk together the garlic, white wine, soy sauce, lemon juice, olive oil, salt and pepper and savory seasoning. Now place the swordfish steaks into the dish and turn them over so that they are coated in the marinade you have just made fully. Then place in the refrigerator for one hour making sure that turn the steaks over frequently during this time.

2. After one hour remove the steaks from the refrigerator and turn on the barbecue. Whilst the barbecue is heating up this will provide the steaks with sufficient time to reach room temperature and so will help to ensure that they then cook properly.

3. As soon as the barbecue has heated up it needs to be as hot as possible you lightly oil the grate and then place the swordfish steaks on to it. Cook for 5 to 6 minutes on each side before then removing to a clean plate and garnish them with some freshly chopped parsley and wedges of lemon.

RECIPE 3 – GRILLED SEA BASS WITH GARLIC SAUCE

If you have never cooked sea bass on a barbecue before this is a very simple and easy recipe that you may want to try. You will find that the garlic butter actually complements the mild flavors of what is a very light and flaky fish.

Ingredients

907grams Sea Bass

3 Tablespoons Butter

1 ½ Tablespoons Extra Virgin Olive Oil

1 Tablespoon Freshly Finely Chopped Italian Parsley

2 Garlic Cloves Minced

¼ Teaspoon Garlic Powder

¼ Teaspoon Paprika

¼ Teaspoon Onion Powder

Lemon Pepper And Salt To Taste

Instructions

1. In a bowl combine together the garlic powder, onion powder, paprika, lemon pepper and salt and then sprinkle this over both sides of the sea bass. Then place in the refrigerator to rest whilst you go ahead and prepare the garlic sauce.

2. To make the garlic sauce into a small saucepan place the butter minced garlic cloves and parsley and heat on a low heat until all the butter has melted. Then place to one side ready to use later on.

3. When it comes to cooking the sea bass on the barbecue you need to do so on a medium high heat and ensure that the grate has been oiled first. Now place the sea bass on the barbecue and cook

it for 7 minutes before then turning it over. After you have turned the fish over brush some of the garlic sauce over the top and then allow the sea bass to cook for a further 7 minutes.

4. As soon as the necessary cooking time has elapsed the fish should flake easily and this is the right time to remove from the heat. Place the fish on a clean plate and then drizzle over some olive oil and some more of the garlic sauce.

RECIPE 4 – BARBECUED SALMON WITH SOY & BROWN SUGAR MARINADE

The mixture of brown sugar, soy sauce, lemon and garlic provides the perfect sweet and salty taste to the rich flavor of the salmon.

Ingredients

700grams Salmon Fillet

1 Tablespoon Lemon Zest

1 Tablespoon Minced Garlic Clove

5 Tablespoons Soy Sauce

4 Tablespoons Dark Brown Soft Sugar

5 Tablespoons Water

4 Tablespoons Vegetable Oil

Freshly Ground Black Pepper To Taste

Instructions

1. In a bowl place the sugar, water, vegetable oil, lemon zest, minced garlic, pepper and soy sauce and mix together until as much of the sugar has dissolved as possible.

2. Once you have made the marinade you now place the salmon fillet into a large resealable plastic bag and pour the marinade over it. Close the bag up and then turn it over several times to ensure that the fillet of salmon is completely covered in the marinade. Place in the refrigerator for at least 2 hours.

3. Once the two hours has passed removed the salmon from the refrigerator and start heating up the barbecue. By the time the barbecue has heated up the salmon fillet should have come up to room temperature and will be ready to start cooking.

4. To cook the salmon fillet on the barbecue you can either place it directly on to the grate that has been lightly oiled or directly on to a piece of aluminum foil that has been lightly oiled. Any marinade that remains should now be discarded.

5. You should cook each side of the salmon for between 5 and 6 minutes or when you use a fork to separate the flesh it flakes easily. Once cooked simply place on a clean plate and then allow your guests to help themselves.

RECIPE 5 – GRILLED ONION BUTTER COD

When cooked on a barbecue you will find the cod becomes very tender and the grilled onion butter enhances not only the flavor but also the texture of this fish. Best served with some grilled potatoes and vegetables.

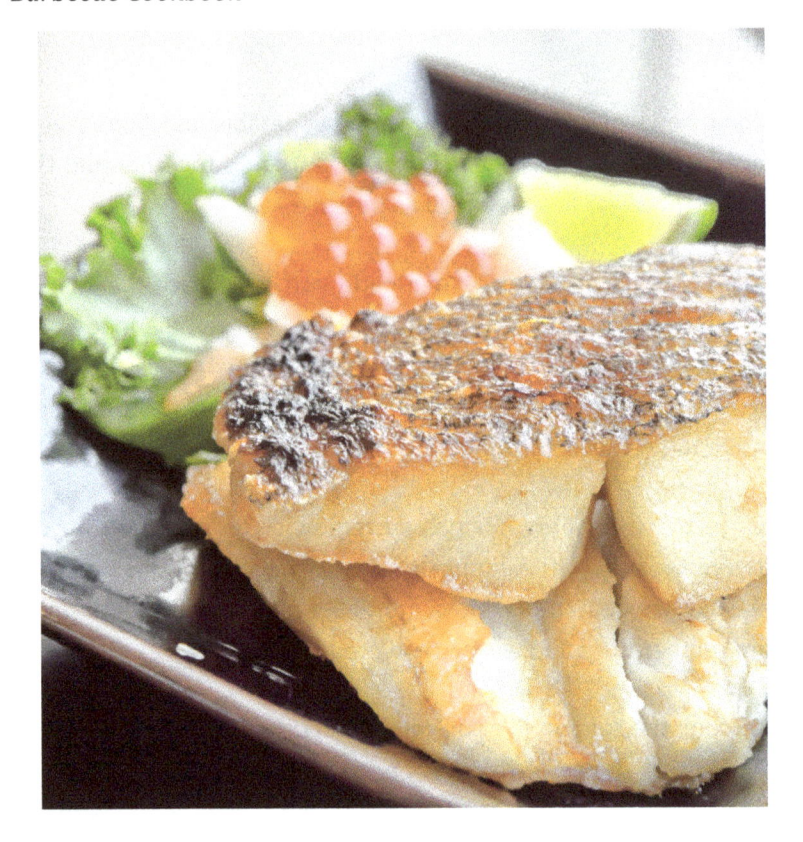

Ingredients

4 Cod Fillets (Each Fillet Should Weigh About 170grams)

1 Small Finely Chopped Onion

60ml White Wine

45gram Butter

1 Tablespoon Extra Virgin Olive Oil

½ Teaspoon Salt

½ Teaspoon Freshly Ground Black Pepper

1 Sliced Lemon

Instructions

1. Whilst the barbecue is heating up you should be preparing the onion butter. To do this into a small frying pan (skillet) place the better and once it is melted to it add the finely chopped onion and allow it to cook for about 1 to 2 minutes. Then to this you add the wine and leave to simmer for 3 minutes. When this time has elapsed remove from the heat and let it cool slightly.

2. As soon as the barbecue has reached the right temperature you should now lightly brush the cod fillets with the olive oil and sprinkle on some salt and black pepper before then placing on to the lightly oiled barbecue grill.

3. Cook the fish on one side for about 8 minutes before then turning it over and basting with some of the butter sauce you made earlier. Now allow the fish to cook for a further 6 to 7 minutes or until you notice the flesh has begun to turn opaque. During this cooking time it is important that you baste the fish with the butter sauce a further 2 or 3 times before then removing from the heat and placing on a clean plate and serving with the wedges of lemon.

RECIPE 6 – GRILLED TROUT WITH PARSLEY

It is best if you use a whole fish rather than fillets as you want to actually place the herbs inside the body of it. You can enjoy this particular barbecue recipe any time of the week.

Ingredients

2 x 450gram Trout (Whole Is Best)

2 Tablespoons Freshly Minced Parsley

2 Tablespoons Olive Oil

2 Tablespoons Freshly Minced Basil

1 Tablespoon Freshly Minced Rosemary

2 Freshly Minced Cloves of Garlic

½ Teaspoon Salt

½ Teaspoon Freshly Ground Black Pepper

Instructions

1. In a small bowl combine together the parsley, olive oil, basil, rosemary and garlic and then spread this evenly over the inside of the fish.

2. Now place the fish in a shallow dish, cover and place in a refrigerator for 2 hours.

3. After 2 hours have elapsed remove the trout from the refrigerator and start heating up the barbecue. Just before placing the trout on to the barbecue grill brush it with some oil and sprinkle both sides of the trout with salt and pepper.

4. Cook the trout on a medium heat for 4 to 5 minutes on each side before carefully removing it and serving the trout on a clean plate.

Recipe 7 – Barbecued Teriyaki Tuna Steaks

Fresh tuna steaks always taste best when cooked on a barbecue. If you want your teriyaki marinade to have a little bit of a kick add some paprika or freshly minced ginger to it.

Samantha Michaels

Ingredients

4 Tuna Steaks (You Can Use Fillets If You Wish)

225ml Teriyaki Sauce

180ml Olive Oil

2 Garlic Cloves Minced

1 Teaspoon Freshly Ground Black Pepper

Instructions

1. Into a large resealable plastic bag pour the teriyaki sauce, olive oil, minced garlic and freshly ground black pepper. Seal the bag up and the shake vigorously to ensure that all these ingredients combine well together.

2. Now place the tuna steaks in the bag and make sure that it is tightly sealed before turning it over several times to ensure that all the marinade coats the steaks well. Now place in the refrigerator to allow the marinade to infuse into the steaks for 30 minutes.

3. Whilst the tuna is in the refrigerator marinating you should now heating up the barbecue. As soon as the barbecue is ready for cooking on take the tuna steaks out of the bag and place them on the oiled barbecue grill and cook until done. If there is any marinade remaining in the bag this should be discarded.

4. As soon as the tuna steaks are cooked remove from barbecue place on clean plates and serve with a fresh crispy green salad.

Recipe 8 – Lime & Basil Tilapia

Combining lime and basil together helps to add even more flavor to the tilapia. You can either serve this barbecue fish dish with some freshly grilled vegetables or you can slice the fish and then serve it in tacos.

Ingredients

4 Tilapia Fillets (Each Weighing Around 115grams)

60ml Olive Oil

2 Tablespoons Lime Juice

Zest of 2 Limes

1 Tablespoon Freshly Minced Basil

2 Teaspoons Bourbon

1 Teaspoon Salt

Freshly Ground Pepper To Taste

Instructions

1. In a resealable plastic bag put the olive oil, lime juice and zest, freshly minced basil, bourbon, salt and pepper. Now close the bag up ensuring it is tightly sealed and shake the contents inside vigorously to make sure that they are all mixed together properly.

2. Once the marinade is prepared you now need to open the bag up and put the tilapia fillets in and seal the bag once more. After

doing this turn the bag over several times to ensure that all of the fillets have been coated in the marinade and then place in a refrigerator for 30 minutes.

3. When the 30 minutes have elapsed remove the fillets from the bag and pour any marinade left in the bag into a saucepan. Whilst the barbecue is heating up you now need to heat the marinade up in the saucepan and then bring it to a low boil. As soon as the marinade starts to boil remove from the heat and place to one side.

4. Next you need to cook the Tilapia fillets. It is important that you cook this fish on a high heat and each side should be cooked for at least 3 minutes. As soon as the fish has turned opaque you should remove it from the heat and serve with some of the marinade in the saucepan drizzled over the top.

RECIPE 9 – BARBECUED TUNA WITH HONEY GLAZE

The lime coriander and honey help to enhance the flavor of what is quite a meaty fish further.

Ingredients

450grams Tuna Fillets

4 Tablespoons Olive Oil

4 Tablespoons Lime Juice (Fresh Would Be Best)

2 Tablespoons Balsamic Vinegar

2 Cloves Garlic Minced

1 Tablespoon Freshly Minced Ginger Root

1 Small Bunch Freshly Chopped Coriander

Honey Glaze

4 Tablespoons Honey

2 Tablespoons Olive Oil

2 Tablespoons Freshly Chopped Coriander

Instructions

1. Into a medium size bowl mix together the olive oil, lime juice, minced garlic, balsamic vinegar, freshly minced ginger root and freshly chopped coriander. Once all these ingredients have been combined well together you add the tuna fillets and turn them over several times to ensure that each one is evenly coated in the marinade. Now cover the bowl over and place in a refrigerator and leave for several hours.

2. After several hours now is the time to start heating up the barbecue. It is important that when cooking the tuna on the barbecue you do so on a high heat. Whilst the barbecue is heating up this is the time when you should be making the honey glaze.

3. To make the honey glaze place the honey, olive oil and freshly chopped coriander in a bowl and whisk. Then set it to one side.

4. By the time you have finished making the honey glaze the barbecue should have reached the desired temperature for cooking the tuna fillets. However before you place the tuna fillets on the grill make sure that you lightly oil it first.

5. Once you have placed the tuna on the grill close the lid and allow the fillets to cook for 1 to 2 minutes before opening the lid and then turning the fillets over. Now close the lid for a further minute then open the lid and continue to cook the tuna until it is barely done. It is important that whilst the tuna fillets are cooking you baste them regularly with the marinade.

6. As soon as the tuna fillets are nearly cooked through you should brush both sides of them with the honey glaze and then remove from the barbecue and serve.

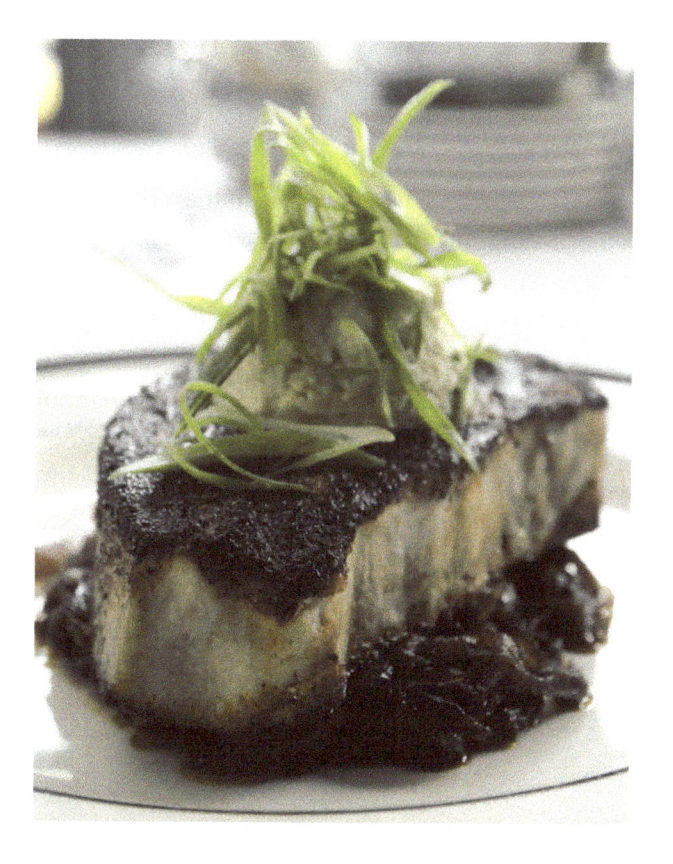

RECIPE 10 – BLACKENED FISH

The great thing about cooking blackened fish on a barbecue is that you won't find your kitchen filling up with smoke.

Ingredients

6 Firm Fish Fillets

3 Tablespoons Cajun Blackening Spices

339grams Unsalted Butter Melted

Instructions

1. Heat up the barbecue until it is good and hot. Once the barbecue has reached the desired temperature now you can begin cooking the fish fillets.

2. Pour most of the melted butter into a shallow dish (leave around 12 tablespoons of the butter to one side as you will use this later when serving the fish). After pouring the melted butter into the dish dip each fillet (both sides) in it before then sprinkling some of the Cajun blackening spices over them.

3. Once this has been done place the fillets on the oiled barbecue grill and cook for about 2 minutes before then turning them over and cooking the other side for a further 2 minutes. As soon as this time has elapsed or when you feel the fillets are cooked through remove from heat and place on clean plates along with a small bowl in which some of the remaining butter has been placed that your guests can then dip the fish fillets into.

RECIPE 11 – CITRUS MARJORAM MARINATED HALIBUT STEAK

It is important that when making the citrus marinade for this particular recipe that you use sprigs of fresh marjoram. Also it is important that you only allow the fish to marinate in the sauce for no more than 2 hours. If you marinate it for any longer than this the texture of the fish will be affected.

Ingredients

800grams Halibut Steaks

7 Tablespoons Fresh Grapefruit Juice

4 Tablespoons Olive Oil

1 Dessertspoon Freshly Chopped Marjoram

½ Teaspoon Salt

1/8 Teaspoon Freshly Ground Black Pepper

4 Springs Fresh Marjoram To Use As Garnish

Instructions

1. In a shallow dish mix together the grapefruit juice, olive oil, freshly chopped marjoram, salt and pepper.

2. To this mixture add the fish making sure you turn it over so both sides are coated in the marinade. Now cover and place in the refrigerator for 1 to 2 hours. Whilst it is marinating make sure that you turn the fish over once or twice.

3. After the marinating time has elapsed you should start heating up the barbecue, with the grill placed 4 to 6 inches above the heat source. Whilst the barbecue is heating up take the fish out of the refrigerator so that they come up to room temperature.

4. When the barbecue has heated up now place the halibut steaks into a fish basket that has been lightly oiled and place on the barbecue grill. You should cook these steaks for between 10 and 12 minutes turning them once and brushing with any marinade you have left over. Serve once the steaks have become barely opaque in the thickest part on a clean plate with the sprigs of fresh marjoram.

RECIPE 12 – GRILLED RED SNAPPER

You will need a whole red snapper for this recipe. But don't worry grilling a whole fish isn't as difficult as it sounds, especially if you have never done it before.

Ingredients

970grams Whole Red Snapper (Split and Butterflied)

60ml Achiote Paste

60ml Orange Juice

3 Tablespoons Lemon Juice

3 Tablespoons Lime Juice

(If you can use fresh orange, lemon and lime juice)

Instructions

1. In a bowl mix together the achiote paste with the orange, lemon and lime juice and spread over all surfaces of the Red Snapper.

Place into a shallow dish which you then cover before putting in the refrigerator to rest for at least 2 hours.

2. Just before the fish comes out of the refrigerator start up the barbecue and place the grill about 6 inches above the heat source as you want to cook this fish on a medium heat.

3. Once the barbecue has heated up lightly oil the grill and then place the Red Snapper on it skin side down and leave it there for about 5 minutes. Then after this time turning the fish over and let it cook for a further 3 minutes. You will notice that the fish is done when the juices begin boiling and also you will find removing the central bone is easy because it simply lifts out when the fish is cooked.

4. If you would like to cook the fish in the same way that Mexican people do then try and get a banana leaf on which to place it when cooking. If you can make sure that the leaf is still wet when you place it on the grill first before adding the fish. Not only will this prevent the fish from sticking to the grill but also help to stop it from falling apart as you turn it over.

RECIPE 13 – GINGER SWORDFISH

An amazing marinade that really helps to bring some amazing flavors out of the swordfish.

Ingredients

6 Swordfish Steaks

175ml Teriyaki Sauce

Barbecue Cookbook

150ml Dry Sherry

8 Garlic Cloves Freshly Minced

1 Dessertspoon Freshly Minced Ginger Root

1 Teaspoon Sesame Oil

Instructions

1. Into a saucepan (large) place the teriyaki sauce, dry sherry, garlic, ginger and sesame oil, mix and bring up to the boil. Once boiling remove the pan from the heat and set to one side to cool for 10 minutes.

2. In a shallow dish place the swordfish steaks and pour some of the marinade over the top that you made earlier. Then turn the steaks over and pour the rest of the marinade over them. Cover the dish up and place in the refrigerator for 1 ½ hours. During this time you should make sure that you turn the Swordfish steaks over frequently.

3. About 15 minutes before you remove the fish from the refrigerator you should get the barbecue started and place the grill about 4 to 6 inches above the heat source. This type of fish should be cooked on a medium to high heat.

4. Once the barbecue has heated up you can now place the steaks on the lightly oiled grill and cook them on each side for 4 minutes. The best way of telling that the Swordfish steaks are cooked is that when prodded with a fork the meat should easily flake. Serve to your guests immediately after removing from the barbecue.

Recipe 14 – Grilled Asian Style Catfish

This is one of the simplest recipes you can use to prepare catfish for cooking on a barbecue. Simply mix together the various ingredients that make up the marinade, place the fish in the marinade and allow it to remain in it for up to 8 hours.

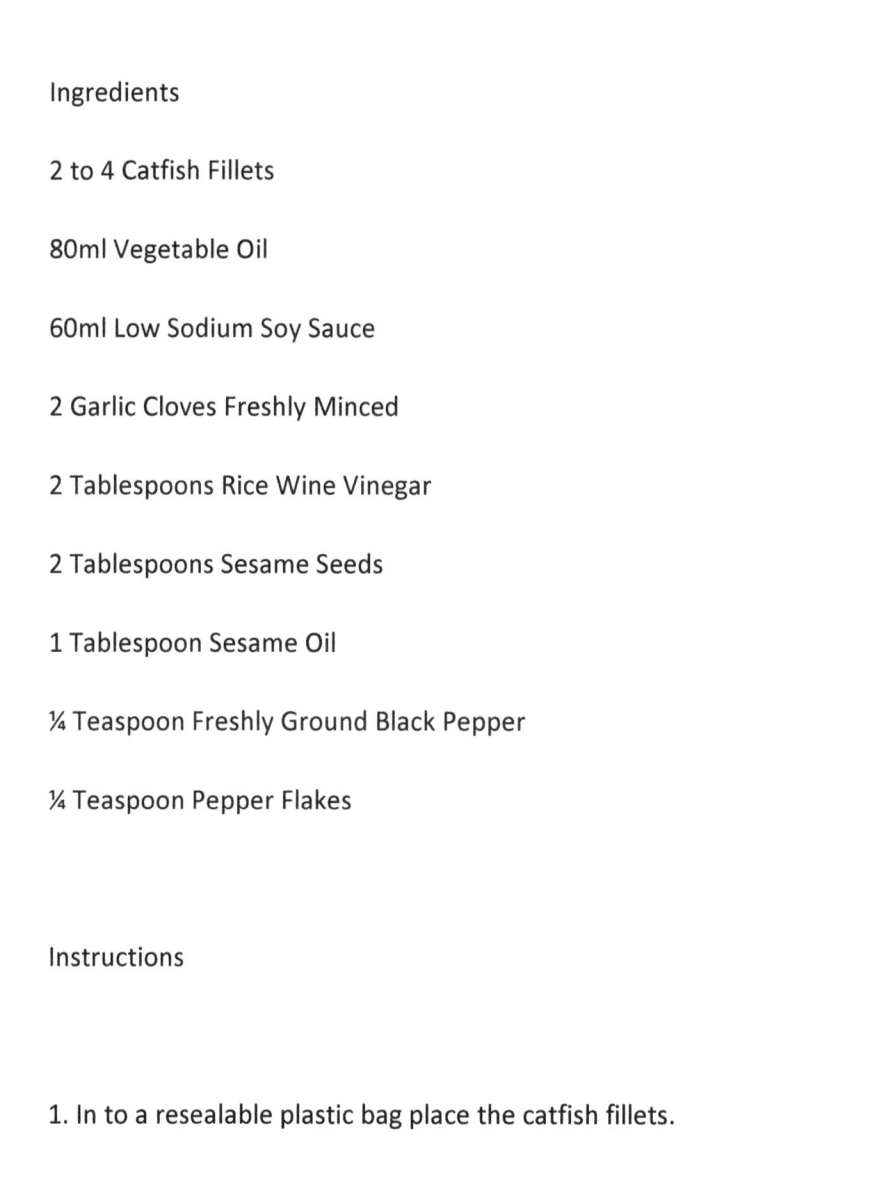

Ingredients

2 to 4 Catfish Fillets

80ml Vegetable Oil

60ml Low Sodium Soy Sauce

2 Garlic Cloves Freshly Minced

2 Tablespoons Rice Wine Vinegar

2 Tablespoons Sesame Seeds

1 Tablespoon Sesame Oil

¼ Teaspoon Freshly Ground Black Pepper

¼ Teaspoon Pepper Flakes

Instructions

1. In to a resealable plastic bag place the catfish fillets.

2. In a small bowl now combine together the vegetable oil, soy sauce, garlic, rice wine vinegar, sesame seeds, sesame oil, black pepper and pepper flakes. Then pour over the fillets in the bag and seal it. Turn the bag over several times to ensure that the catfish fillets have been well coated in the marinade before then placing the bag in the refrigerator and leaving there for 1 to 8 hours. The longer you let the fish remain in the marinade the more of its flavor will be absorbed by the fish.

3. As soon as you are ready to cook the fish then heat up the barbecue and make sure that you place the grill at a height that allows you to cook the catfish fillets on a medium to high heat.

4. Once the barbecue has heated up remove the catfish fillets from the marinade, which can now be discarded and place the fillets on the grill, which you have lightly oiled first and cook for between 12 and 13 minutes. During this time you must turn the fillets over at least once. The fish will be cooked when it easily flakes with a fork. As soon as the fish is cooked remove from heat and serve to your guests.

RECIPE 15 – BARBECUED SEA BASS

This is a very simple barbecue recipe for cooking sea bass. However it is best if at possible to use as fresh a fish as possible. Not only perfect for cooking at home but also at the beach.

Ingredients

500gram Fresh Sea Bass

1 Tablespoon Fresh Lemon Juice

Samantha Michaels

1 Teaspoon Olive Oil

Salt & Freshly Ground Black Pepper To Taste

1 Bay Leaf

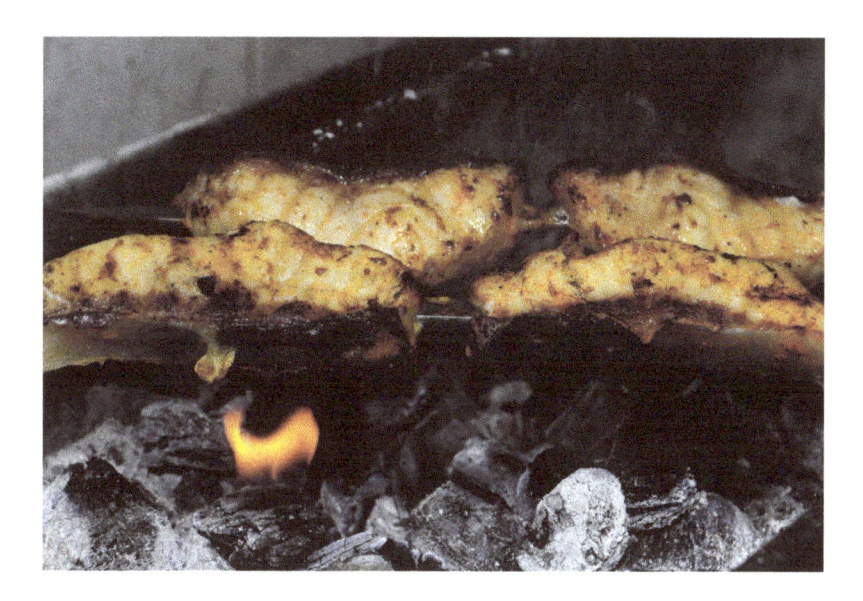

Instructions

1. In a bowl mix together the lemon juice, olive oil, salt, pepper and bay leaf. Then rub the sea bass both inside and out with this. You should be doing this whilst the barbecue is heating up.

2. As soon as the barbecue has heated up place the fish on the lightly oiled grilled about 4 to 6 inches above the heat source and cook for around 8 to 10 minutes. Halfway through the cooking time you should turn the fish over and finish off cooking. You will know when the fish is cooked as it flakes easily with a fork.

Recipe 16 – Grilled Trout In Corn Husks

This is a recipe that will impress your guests and also is a very quick and easy way to prepare and serve trout to them.

Ingredients

4 Trout Fillets

4 Fresh Corn Husks

8 Strips Bacon

20grams Unsalted Butter

½ Teaspoon Freshly Ground Black Pepper

Kitchen Twine

Instructions

1. Check the fish over to make sure that there are no bones in the fillets. Whilst you are doing this now is the time to get the barbecue heated up.

2. Once you have checked to make sure there are no more bones in the fish you can now start making up the little corn husk packets. Place a fillet on each corn husk and then over these place two of the slices of bacon along with 5 grams of the butter. Now close the husks up and secure them in place by wrapping some of the kitchen twine around them.

3. Once you have placed the twine around the corn husks you can place the packets on to the barbecue grill and cook for between 15

and 18 minutes or until the fish is cooked through. As soon as the fish is ready remove from heat and serve to your guests with barbecued corn on the cob and some fresh new potatoes.

RECIPE 17 – GRILLED JAMAICAN JERK CATFISH

Although relatively spicy you can add a little more of kick to yours if want by adding an additional freshly chopped jalapeno in to the seasoning mixture.

Ingredients

4 Catfish Fillets

2 Green Onions Finely Chopped

1 Jalapeno Pepper Seeded And Chopped

2 Tablespoons Brown Sugar

2 Tablespoons Worcestershire Sauce

2 Tablespoons White Wine Vinegar

1 Tablespoon Freshly Minced Ginger

1 Garlic Clove Minced

1 Teaspoon Allspice

½ Teaspoon Dried Thyme

¼ Teaspoon Salt

1/8 Teaspoon Freshly Ground Black Pepper

Instructions

1. Preheat heat the barbecue to a medium heat. Whilst the barbecue is heating up in to a bowl (large) place the onions, jalapeno pepper, brown sugar, Worcestershire sauce, white wine vinegar, ginger, garlic, allspice, dried thyme, salt and pepper and mix thoroughly.

2. Now into the bowl add the fish and coat well before then covering the bowl and leaving the fish to marinate in the sauce for 5 to 10 minutes at room temperature.

3. After the relevant amount of time has elapsed remove the catfish fillets from the marinade and place them to one side. Don't throw away the marinade as you are going to need this.

4. Place the catfish fillets on the barbecue grill that has been lightly oiled and brush with some of the remaining marinade. Now cook for about 5 minutes before then turning the fish over. After turning the fish over you need to again brush with the marinade that is remaining and cook for a further 7 to 9 minutes. As soon as the fillets are cooked remove from the barbecue and serve with a crisp fresh green salad.

Recipe 18 – Grilled Tandoori Cod

As well as being very easy to prepare you will find that this particular recipe tastes absolutely delicious. Serve either with some freshly grilled vegetables or with some rice.

Ingredients

4 to 6 Cod Fillets Cut Into ½ Inch Chunks

240ml Plain Yogurt

Samantha Michaels

60ml Olive Oil

4 Garlic Cloves Minced

2 Teaspoons Freshly Grated Ginger

2 Teaspoons Ground Cumin

2 Teaspoons Ground Coriander

1 Teaspoon Red Pepper

1 Teaspoon Turmeric

1 Teaspoon Salt

Instructions

1. In a medium size bowl combine together the yogurt, olive oil, garlic, ginger, cumin, coriander, red pepper, turmeric and salt. Once combined together well add the chunks of cod and mix again. It is important to make sure that every piece of cod is coated well in the marinade you have just made.

2. Now cover the bowl over and place in a refrigerator for 1 hour to let the fish absorb as much of the marinade as possible.

3. About 15 minutes before you remove the fish from the refrigerator you should now start heating up your barbecue. Put the grill at a height of about 4 to 6 inches above the heat source so that the fish will then cook on a medium to high heat.

4. As soon as the barbecue has heated up sufficiently you are now ready to start cooking the fish. Remove the fish from the marinade and thread on to wooden skewers that have been soaking in water

for around 30 minutes and then place them on to the lightly oiled grill.

Cook for around 17 to 19 minutes turning frequently to ensure that the fish doesn't get burnt. When the flesh of the code turns opaque you can now remove from the heat and serve.

RECIPE 19 – GRILLED MUSTARD & MISO SEA BASS

This particular recipe requires you to use white miso paste that is much sweeter and milder than the dark versions. When you allow the sea bass to marinade in the miso, rice wine and mustard sauce it help to make the fish much more tender and taste more delicious.

Ingredients

4 Sea Bass Fillets each weighing About 140 to 170grams

6 Green Onions Trimmed

80ml White Miso Paste

3 Tablespoons Rice Vinegar

2 Tablespoons Japanese Rice Wine (Mirin)

2 Tablespoons Toasted Sesame Seeds

3 Teaspoons Sugar

2 Teaspoons Water

1 Garlic Clove Minced

1 Teaspoon Dijon Mustard

1 Teaspoon Soy Sauce

Olive Oil

Salt

Freshly Ground Black Pepper

Instructions

1. Whilst the barbecue is heating up in to a bowl mix together the water and mustard until they are mixed thoroughly.

2. Now into a small saucepan place the miso, vinegar, mirin, soy sauce, garlic, sugar and mustard mixture and place pan on to a medium heat. Whisk the mixture whilst heating until it turns smooth, this should take between 3 to 5 minutes to happen. Once the mixture has turned smooth remove from heat and brush the sauce over the fish and also brush the green onions with some olive oil. Sprinkle the fish and onions with salt and pepper to taste.

3. Now place the fish on to the barbecue grill which has been lightly oiled and cook on either side for 4 to 5 minutes or the flesh inside turns opaque in color.

4. Next you need to cook the fish for a further 2 minutes on either side and whilst this is happening you should place the green onions on the grill to cook as well.

You are now ready to remove the fish and onions from the barbecue to serve to your guests. Place each fish on a clean plate with the onions and a small amount of the miso sauce you have left over and sprinkle over some of the toasted sesame seeds.

RECIPE 20 – SEA BASS KEBABS

If you want to prepare sea bass quickly and easily this is the perfect barbecue recipe to use. They are suitable for any kind of barbecue party you are going to be having.

Ingredients

680grams Sea Bass Cut Into ½ Inch Chunks

60ml Fresh Lemon Juice

60ml Olive Oil

2 Garlic Cloves Minced

1 Teaspoon Dried Oregano

¼ Teaspoon Salt

¼ Teaspoon Freshly Ground Black Pepper

Instructions

1. In a large bowl mix together the lemon juice, olive oil, garlic, oregano, salt and pepper. Once thoroughly combined together add in the chunks of sea bass and then cover the bowl and place in the refrigerator to marinate for 1 to 2 hours.

2. About 15 minutes before you remove the sea bass from the refrigerator you should start warming up the barbecue. You will need to cook the kebabs on a very high heat. If you are going to be using wooden skewers then make sure that these have been

soaking in water for no less than an hour, as this will then prevent them from burning when placed on the barbecue.

3. As you remove each piece of fish from the marinade thread them on to the skewers and place to one side ready for cooking. Don't discard any left over marinade, as you will be using this later on when cooking the fish.

4. As soon as the barbecue is hot enough you can place the kebabs on the grill. Make sure that you have lightly oiled the grill first to prevent the fish kebabs from sticking to it and cook them for between 5 and 7 minutes. As well as turning the kebabs over frequently to prevent them from burning also baste them with any marinade that is left over. As soon as the kebabs are ready serve.

Recipe 21 – Grilled Thai Red Snapper Packets

This recipe allows you to cook red snapper on your barbecue without leaving any mess to clear up afterwards.

Ingredients

4 Red Snapper Fillets (140 to 170grams)

1 Carrot Julienne

1 Green Onion Minced

32grams Fresh Cilantro

3 Tablespoons Fresh Lime Juice

2 Garlic Cloves Minced

1 Tablespoon Fish Sauce

1 Tablespoon Olive Oil

1 Teaspoon Freshly Minced Ginger

Aluminum Foil

Instructions

1. Start the barbecue is up so it is ready for placing the packets containing the red snapper on to cook.

2. Whilst the barbecue is heating up in a small bowl mix together the fish sauce, olive oil, ginger, lime juice, sugar and garlic.

3. On to four separate pieces of aluminum foil you place one of the four red snapper fillets (skin side down) and pour over some of the mixture you have just made. Then sprinkle over the top of this some of the carrots, cilantro and green onion. Then bring up the sides of the aluminum to seal the fish inside. But don't secure the packets too tightly as you need to allow some of the steam produced as the fish cooks to escape.

4. As soon as the barbecue has heated up place the Thai red snapper packets on the grill and cook for between 8 and 10 minutes. Once this time has elapsed remove from the barbecue and then cut open the packets with a pair of scissors and serve without removing them from the aluminum foil on a clean plate.

Recipe 22 – Moroccan Grilled Fish Kebabs

This is very simple dish to prepare but provides the fish you use with lots of flavor.

Ingredients

680grams White Fish Fillets Cut Into Chunks

32grams Red Onion Chopped

80ml Olive Oil

2 Tablespoons Fresh Cilantro Finely Chopped

3 Tablespoons Fresh Lemon Juice

½ Teaspoon Paprika

½ Teaspoon Salt

¼ Teaspoon Freshly Ground Black Pepper

¼ Teaspoon Chilli Powder

2 Garlic Cloves Minced

Wooden Skewers which have been soaked in water for at least 30 minutes.

Instructions

1. Cut the fillets of fish into chunks measuring an inch each and place them in a resealable plastic bag.

2. Now in to a bowl place the onion, olive oil, cilantro, lemon juice, paprika, salt, pepper, chilli powder and minced garlic and stir well to ensure that the ingredients are mixed thoroughly together. Now pour this mixture into the same bag as the fish. Then close the bag and turn it over or shake until all pieces of fish have been coated in the marinade you have just made. Once you have done this place the sealed bag in to a refrigerator and leave there for between 2 and 4 hours.

3. When it comes to cooking the fish remove from the bag discarding any marinade that remains and thread each chunk of fish on to the skewers you have been soaking in water. Once you have thread each skewer with fish you should now lightly oil the grill on your preheated barbecue and place the skewers on to it.

You should be cooking the fish kebabs on a medium to high heat for between 8 and 10 minutes making sure that you turn them over occasionally to prevent them from burning. As soon as they have cooked you should remove them from the barbecue and serve to your guests immediately.

Recipe 23 – Grilled Fish Cakes

It is possible to cook fish cakes on a grill but you do need to be careful when doing so.

Ingredients

450grams White Fish Fillets

1 Onion Chopped

6 Cashew Nuts

1 Teaspoon Chili Powder

½ Teaspoon Tumeric

1 Tablespoon Freshly Chopped Lemon Grass

1 Teaspoon Freshly Chopped Mint

½ Teaspoon Freshly Grated Black Pepper

1 Tablespoon Sugar

120ml Coconut Milk

1 Tablespoon Coriander

Salt To Taste

Banana Leafs For Cooking The Fish Cakes In

Instructions

1. The first thing you should do before you cut the fish fillets into small pieces is to make sure that there no bones inside them.

2. After cutting the fish fillets into small pieces mix them together with the onion, nuts, chili powder, turmeric, lemon grass, mint, black pepper, sugar, coconut milk, coriander and salt in a food processor until they form a smooth mixture.

3. Before you can place any of the fish cake mixture on to a piece of banana leaf measuring 6 inches square they leaves need to be boiled in water for about a minute as this will help to soften them up and make them more pliable to use. As soon as the banana leaves are ready place 2 tablespoons of the fish cake mixture on to each one and then fold the leaves over. To keep the leaves securely

in place pierce through the areas where they come together with a toothpick. You should be doing this whilst the barbecue is heating up.

4. As soon as the barbecue has heated place the banana leaves with the fish cake mixture inside on to the barbecue and cook on a high heat for 5 minutes. It is important that halfway through this time you turn the fish cakes over to ensure that they are cooked evenly. Once the fish cakes are ready serve to your guests still encased in the banana leaves.

RECIPE 24 – TARRAGON FISH WITH VEGETABLES

Wrapping up the fish with the vegetables and tarragon help to add more flavor to this dish. Plus you won't make as much mess when cooking them because the fish and other ingredients are wrapped up.

Ingredients

2 x 170grams Fish Fillets (You May Want To Give Orange Roughy A Try)

½ Zucchini Cut Into Julienne Strips

½ Small Red Bell Pepper Cut Into Thin Strips

32grams Sliced Red Onion

1 Carrot Cut Into Julienne Strips

1 Tablespoon Canola Oil

2 Tablespoons Freshly Chopped Tarragon (If you cannot get hold of fresh tarragon use ¾ Teaspoon of Dried Tarragon Instead)

1 Tablespoon Butter

Instructions

1. Whilst the barbecue is heating up in a frying pan place the oil and cook the vegetables for about 2 to 3 minutes on a medium to high heat. Then place to one side, as you will need them in a minute.

2. Next take too large pieces of aluminum foil and on to these place the fish fillets then on top of these place ½ tablespoon of the butter, half the vegetables and half of the tarragon. Then tightly wrap the foil around each piece and place on the grill of the barbecue.

3. Grill each piece of fish on a medium heat for between 12 and 18 minutes. How long you cook them for will depend on how thick each fish fillet is. The thicker the fillet then the longer they will need to remain on the barbecue.

It is important that after removing the packets from the barbecue that you open them carefully as the steam released can be extremely hot and can cause burns.

RECIPE 25 – ITALIAN STYLE TROUT

The stuffing of the trout with the olives and shallots adds even more flavor to what is a very tasty fish. Make sure that you cook these on a very high heat and don't allow them to remain on the barbecue for too long.

Ingredients

4 Trout (Heads Removed, Boned And Butterflied)

4 Tablespoons Butter

32grams Black Olives Which Have Been Coarsely Chopped

2 Tablespoons Pernod (Or Other Liquorice Flavored Liqueur)

2 Tablespoons Olive Oil

1 Tablespoon Freshly Chopped Parsley

1 Small Chopped Shallot

1 Teaspoon Salt

1 Teaspoon Freshly Chopped Chives

½ Teaspoon Freshly Ground Black Pepper

1/8 Teaspoon Freshly Ground Black Pepper

Instructions

1. Sprinkle both sides of the fish with the salt, ½ teaspoon black pepper and Pernod. Now cover and leave the fish to stand for around 30 minutes at room temperature. Whilst this is happening now would be a good time to get the barbecue started.

2. Whilst the fish is left to one side you now need to make up the mixture, which you will then stuff the fish fillets with. In a food processor place the shallots and olives and process them until they are finely chopped. Now to this mixture add the butter, chives, parsley and the 1/8 teaspoon freshly ground black pepper and

again turn the food processor on to blend all these ingredients together well. Once the mixture is ready stuff it inside the fillets of trout and fold the opening closed. If you want you can prevent the fillet from opening again by securing it with a toothpick.

3. As soon as the barbecue has heated up place the trout fillets on to the grill and cook on a medium to high heat for 8 minutes on each side. As soon as the cooking time has been completed remove from heat and serve to your guests on clean plates with a crisp fresh green salad.

RECIPE 26 – PERCH WITH SAGE

This is a really wonderful little recipe to try if you want to grill several perch at once.

Ingredients

2 x 340grams Perch (Scaled)

2 Slices of Zucchini

3 Roma Tomatoes

1 Tablespoon Olive Oil

10 Sprigs of Fresh Sage

Instructions

1. Whilst the barbecue is heating up make around 4 slits into the flesh of the perch on each side. Now coat them with oil and insert sprigs of sage into them.

2. Once the barbecue has heated up place the perch on to the oiled grill and cook for around 4 minutes on each side. As you are about to turn the fish over you should now add the zucchini and tomatoes on to the grill and cook these.

3. As soon as everything has cooked remove everything from the barbecue. To serve the fish remove the sprigs of sage and then stuff them with the tomatoes and zucchini.

RECIPE 27 – SWEET & SOUR HALIBUT

The rich thick sauce that you will eventually pour over the halibut steaks is the same one that you marinated the fish in originally. However it is best to reserve some of the marinate to make the sauce as you don't want it to become contaminated by the fish. This sauce provides the halibut steaks with a great deal of flavor without being too much hassle to create.

Ingredients

4 x Halibut Steaks (Weighing About 340grams Each)

1 Red and Green Bell Pepper

2 Green Onions Cut Into 2 Inch Strips

60ml Water

55grams Brown Sugar

3 Tablespoons Cider Vinegar

3 Tablespoons Tomato Ketchup

1 Tablespoon Soy Sauce

2 Garlic Cloves Minced

¾ Teaspoon Freshly Grated Ginger

Instructions

1. Coat the grill on your barbecue with oil and then turn it on so it can start heating up.

2. Take the bell peppers and cut them in half and remove the seeds then set to one side for use later on.

3. In to bowl place the brown sugar, water, cider vinegar, tomato ketchup, soy sauce, garlic and ginger and mix well together. Remove around 60ml of the sauce you have just made and set aside for later.

4. With the rest of the sauce you have just made dip each of the halibut steaks into it making sure that both sides of the fish have been evenly coated in it and again set to one side.

5. By now the grill should have heated up and you should place the bell peppers on them to cook. Place the peppers on the grill with the skin side down and cook until the skin begins to blacken. Remove once the skin starts to blacken and peel it away from the rest of the pepper. Once the skin has been removed cut them peppers into thin strips.

6. Now place the halibut steaks on the grill and cook until they are done the flesh should start to turn opaque in color. Once the steaks

are cooked place each one on a clean plate then top with some of the slices of the bell peppers and the green onions before then pouring over equal amounts of the sauce that you put aside earlier.

Recipe 28 – Halibut & Red Pepper Kebabs

Halibut is one of the least expensive fishes you can buy today. However by putting the fish onto skewers with peppers and onions you can ensure that you are able to feed more people with only a small amount of the fish.

Ingredients

680grams Halibut Steaks Cut Into 1 Inch Chunks

1 Large Bell Pepper Cut Into 1 Inch Squares

1 Large Red Onion Cut Into 1 Inch Squares

120ml Fresh Lime Juice

4 Tablespoons Olive Oil

3 Tablespoons Fresh Finely Chopped Cilantro

2 Tablespoons Sugar

1 ½ Teaspoons Serrano Pepper Minced (It is important that you wear gloves when dealing with this type of pepper)

Instructions

1. In a small bowl place the lime juice, 2 tablespoons of olive oil, sugar, Serrano pepper and the sugar and combine well together until all the sugar has dissolved. Now leave this to one side for around an hour so that all the flavors blend together.

2. Whilst the sauce is blending you should now be turning the barbecue on so that it can heat up ready to start cooking the halibut, pepper and onion kebabs.

3. To make the kebabs you should thread on to each one alternate pieces of the halibut, pepper and onion until they are all used up. Metal skewers can be used however if you intend to use wooden ones make sure that they have been soaking in some water for at least an hour to ensure that they don't burn when placed on the barbecue.

4. Before you place the kebabs on the grill brush them all over with the remaining olive oil and cook on a high heat for about 1 ½ minutes on all sides so you should be cooking them for a total of around 6 minutes. You will know that the halibut is cooked as it will have turned opaque and will be flaky through the middle.

5. After removing the kebabs from the grill onto a clean plate now serve them with the sauce you made earlier alongside.

RECIPE 29 – FISH ROLL UPS

A very traditional Australian recipe you may want to try out this summer.

Barbecue Cookbook

Ingredients

100grams Smoked Fish

240ml Milk

6 Slices of Buttered Bread

22grams Grated Cheese

3 Tablespoons Butter

3 Tablespoons Flour

1 Teaspoon Lemon Juice (Fresh Is Best)

1 Teaspoon Freshly Chopped Parsley

½ Teaspoon Worcestershire Sauce

¼ Teaspoon Salt

¼ Teaspoon Freshly Ground Black Pepper

Instructions

1. Whilst the barbecue is heating up flake the smoked fish and melt the butter in a saucepan to which you then add the flour, pepper, salt and parsley. Cook this mixture until it begins to boil then very slowly add the milk and then continue cook for a further two minutes. Now add the Worcestershire sauce, cheese, lemon juice and the flaked smoked fish. Mix all the ingredients together well.

2. Now take this mixture and spread it over the unbuttered side of the bread and roll each one up and secure them using a toothpick.

3. Once you have made up each fish roll place them on the barbecue grill, which you can lightly oil, and cook for around 2 to 3 minutes. During this time make sure that you turn them over once and then serve immediately to your waiting guests.

RECIPE 30 – GRILLED SNAPPER IN A BANANA LEAF

This particular method of cooking not only helps to keep the fish together but also helps to steam it to perfection, but still allows some of the smoky flavor to permeate through to the fish also. Plus this method also allows you to add anything you want to the packet to bring out the flavor of the fish even more.

Ingredients

900grams Snapper

2 Tablespoons Freshly Chopped Coriander Root

1 ½ Tablespoons Soy Sauce

1 Tablespoon Freshly Crushed Ginger

2 Garlic Cloves Minced

1 Teaspoon Freshly Ground Black Pepper

Vegetable Oil

Banana Leaf

String

… Barbecue Cookbook

Instructions

1. Into a food processor place the garlic, ginger, black pepper and coriander root and blend together so that it forms a paste. Then add the soy sauce and continue to blend until all the ingredients become well combined. Now set this mixture to one side.

2. Next you should rinse the snapper and then pat it dry with some paper towels. Once you have done this take the sauce you made earlier and rub it all over the surface of the fish and place the fish to one side for 30 minutes. It is now that you should be starting your barbecue up so that it has reached the required temperature for cooking the fish on.

3. Once the 30 minutes have elapsed take the snapper and place it on to the banana leaf. It is important that the leaves you use are large enough to completely cover the fish. However if you cannot get large ones then it is perfectly to cut the fish into pieces that will fit easily inside the leaves you do have.

But before you do wrap the fish in the leaves make sure that you have washed them thoroughly. Also they need to be blanched in hot water for a number of seconds as this will help to make the soft and so much easier to wrap around the fish.

After the banana leaves have been blanched you should remove the thick spine from them with a pair of kitchen scissors. Then place them on a work surface shiny side facing downwards.

Then you must brush vegetable oil all over the leaf facing towards you, which will then come into contact with the fish. Once you have done this you can place the fish on to and then wrap the leaf around it. To help keep the leaf around the fish when cooking secure it in place either with a skewer or toothpicks.

4. After wrapping the snapper in the banana leaf you can now place it on the barbecue to cook. Cook it on a medium heat so

place the grill around 4 to 6 inches above the heat source and cook on each side for between 8 and 10 minutes. You need to keep an eye on the fish as it is cooking to ensure that the banana leaf doesn't become burnt. Although it may start to blacken in areas you don't want the heat to burn right through the leaf.

5. After 16 minutes remove the packages from the barbecue and very gently open them to see whether the fish is cooked or not. You will know when the fish is cooked because it is opaque in appearance and flakes easily with a fork. If you notice that the fish isn't cooked then securely wrap back in the banana leaf and place on the barbecue again for another couple of minutes.

When it comes to serving this dish it is best to allow the fish to remain enclosed in the banana leaf and open it when you reach the table.

Recipe 31 – South Western Mahi Mahi

This is the perfect recipe to use if you want to serve Mexican style food for your guests at your next barbecue. You can use this particular recipe to make some amazing fish tacos.

Ingredients

6 x 170grams Mahi Mahi Fish Fillets (If you cannot get hold of this fish then use Halibut fillets instead)

40grams Freshly Chopped Cilantro

60ml Fresh Lemon Juice

2 Tablespoons Olive Oil

1 Tablespoon Honey

3 Garlic Cloves Minced

1 Teaspoon Hot Chilli Powder (Optional)

Salt and Freshly Ground Black Pepper To Taste

Instructions

1. In a bowl combine well together the cilantro, lemon juice, olive oil, honey, garlic, salt and pepper. Plus the hot chilli powder if you want to add a little kick to this dish. Then set to one side.

2. Now into a resealable bag or on a shallow baking dish place the fish fillets and pour over the sauce you made earlier.

Remember to turn the fish over so that all sides are coated in the marinade and leave if the refrigerator to marinate for 30 minutes. Whilst the fish is marinating in the refrigerator you should be lighting your barbecue so that it is ready then for cooking the fish once you take it out of the refrigerator.

3. To cook the fish remove from the marinade and place on the barbecue directly over the heat sauce and then cook on each side for 3 to 4 minutes or until the fish is cooked through. To check to see if it is done see if the fish flakes easily with a fork and has turned opaque through out.

Recipe 32 – Grilled Shark

Shark actually has a great flavor and the sauce in which you marinate the fish helps to enhance rather than overpower its flavor.

Ingredients

6 Shark Steaks

120ml Soy Sauce

60ml Tomato Ketchup

120ml Fresh Orange Juice

40grams Freshly Chopped Parsley

2 Tablespoons Fresh Lemon Juice

2 Garlic Cloves Minced

1/3 Tablespoon Freshly Ground Pepper

Instructions

1. In a bowl combine together the garlic, pepper, soy sauce, orange juice, tomato ketchup, chopped parsley and lemon juice.

2. Take the shark steaks and place them in a shallow baking dish and pour the sauce you have just made over them. It is important that you turn the steaks over to ensure that all sides of them are coated in the sauce, which you are going to be marinating them in. Now cover the dish and place in the refrigerator for 2 hours.

3. When it comes time to cook the shark steaks make sure that the grill on the barbecue has been lightly oiled first to prevent them from sticking to the surface. As soon as the barbecue has heated up remove the steaks from the marinate and place them on the grill keeping any left over marinate in the dish for use later.

4. Grill the shark steaks over a high heat for 6 minutes on each side or until when tested with a fork the fish flakes easily. Throughout the time the shark steaks are cooking make sure that you baste them regularly with the remainder of the sauce you marinated them in earlier.

RECIPE 33 – GRILLED CATFISH

Not only is this a quick and easy way to cook catfish. But adding the sauce whilst cooking adds even more flavor to it.

Ingredients

450grams Catfish Fillet

3 Garlic Cloves Crushed

2 Tablespoons Lemon Juice (Fresh If Possible)

1 Tablespoon Balsamic Vinegar

1 Teaspoon Soy Sauce

2 Sprigs Fresh Rosemary

1 Teaspoon Cayenne Pepper

Instructions

1. Whilst the barbecue is heating up place the catfish fillet on to a piece of aluminum foil that is large enough that when you fold the edges up it turns into a makeshift pan.

2. Now place the fish in the aluminum foil on to the barbecue and them pour over the other ingredients and let the catfish fillet cook them until it is done. On average the fish should be cooked in about 4 to 9 minutes depending on how hot the barbecue is and what the weather is like. It is important that you watch the fish carefully whilst it is cooking otherwise it could become over cooked very easily.

You will know when the fish is cooked because the edges of it start to turn up and become crispy. But don't rely on this solely for telling you that the fish is cooked you should check to see if the middle of the catfish fillet has turned opaque.

RECIPE 34 – SPICY TUNA STEAKS

When it comes to cooking tuna steaks on a barbecue make sure that you do so on a very high heat. Also use the best quality steaks you can, as these will only require warming through to the middle.

Ingredients

6 Small Tuna Steaks (Weighing Around 170grams Each)

80ml Olive Oil

80ml Lemon Juice (Fresh Would Be Best)

Barbecue Cookbook

4 Tablespoons Chopped Cilantro Leaves

3 Garlic Cloves Minced

3 Shallots Minced

2 Teaspoons Cayenne Pepper

2 Teaspoons Ground Cumin

1 Teaspoon Salt

Instructions

1. In a bowl combine together well the lemon juice, olive oil, and 3 tablespoons of the cilantro leaves, garlic, shallots, cumin, cayenne pepper and salt.

2. Now into a large resealable bag you place the tuna steaks and then pour the sauce you have just made over them. Make sure that you turn the bag over several times to ensure the sauce coats the steaks evenly then place in the refrigerator for 1 hour to allow them to marinate in the sauce.

3. About 15 minutes before you remove the tuna steaks from the refrigerator you should start up your barbecue so it is heated up correctly for cooking the steaks on it.

4. Just before you take the steaks out of the marinade after removing from the refrigerator lightly oil the grill on your barbecue and then place the tuna steaks on them. Make sure the grill is placed as close to the heat source as possible as you need to cook the steaks on a high heat.

5. You should cook each side of the tuna steaks for around 4 to 5 minutes or until you feel they are cooked to the way people enjoy

eating this type of fish. Once they are cooked remove from the barbecue place on clean plates and sprinkle with the remaining cilantro and then serve.

RECIPE 35 – ASIAN JERK RED SNAPPER

As well as using jerk seasoning this particular recipe also uses an Asian style baste to help bring out even more of the wonderful flavor of this particular fish.

Ingredients

2 Whole Red Snapper (Weighing About 900grams Each)

4 Green Onions Diced

4 Garlic Cloves Minced

60ml Lemon Juice

Zest Of Two Lemons

2 Tablespoons Jerk Rub

2 Tablespoons Olive Oil

2 Tablespoons Soy Sauce

Instructions

1. In a small bowl combine together 2 minced garlic cloves, scallions, lemon zest and 1 tablespoon Jerk rub. Then rub it all over the insides of the cleaned out red snapper.

2. Now into another bowl you should combine together the other 1 tablespoon jerk rub along with the rest of the garlic, the lemon juice, the soy sauce and olive oil and place to one side. It is important that before you start making up the above you actually turn the barbecue on so it will then be ready for cooking the fish on.

3. As soon as the barbecue has heated up place the red snapper on to the grill about 4 to 6 inches above the heat source so it cooks on a medium to high heat. Let the fish cook on each side for 8 to 10 minutes and whilst this is happening baste frequently with the lemon, soy sauce and jerk rub sauce.

RECIPE 36 – GRILLED FRESH SARDINES

This recipe helps to turn what is quite a humble fish into something a little special. Plus it is also good for your health as it helps to reduce "bad cholesterol" levels.

Ingredients

8 Medium Sized Whole Fresh Sardines

(These should be gutted, and then rinsed inside and out before then being patted dry with a paper towel).

1 ½ Tablespoons Extra Virgin Olive Oil

¾ Teaspoon Coarse Salt

¼ Teaspoon Freshly Ground Black Pepper

1 Garlic Clove Peeled

6 Inch Baguette Cut Into 16 Thin Slices Diagonally

Instructions

1. Brush both sides of the sardines with 1 tablespoon of the extra virgin olive oil and thin sprinkle over them 1/2 teaspoon of salt and 1/8 teaspoon of the freshly ground black pepper. Whilst you are doing this heat up the barbecue.

2. Once the barbecue is hot enough lightly oil the surface of the grill and them place the sardines on to it and cook them on a medium to high heat. Cook each sardine for 2 minutes on each side.

3. Halfway through cooking the sardines you should also be cooking the slices of baguette that you will be serving with the fish.

But before placing the baguette slices on the barbecue first rub each side of them with the garlic and brush them with the rest of the olive oil. Then sprinkle with the salt and pepper that is left over. Cook each side of the bread for 1 minute or until they turn crisp.

4. As soon as everything is cooked place the sardines and bread on to a clean plate and serve with some lemon wedges to your guests.

Barbecue Cookbook

Recipe 37 – Grilled Squid With Ginger, Celery & Apple Salad

This really does give a kick to this particular recipe and also helps to counteract some of the heat generated by the ginger.

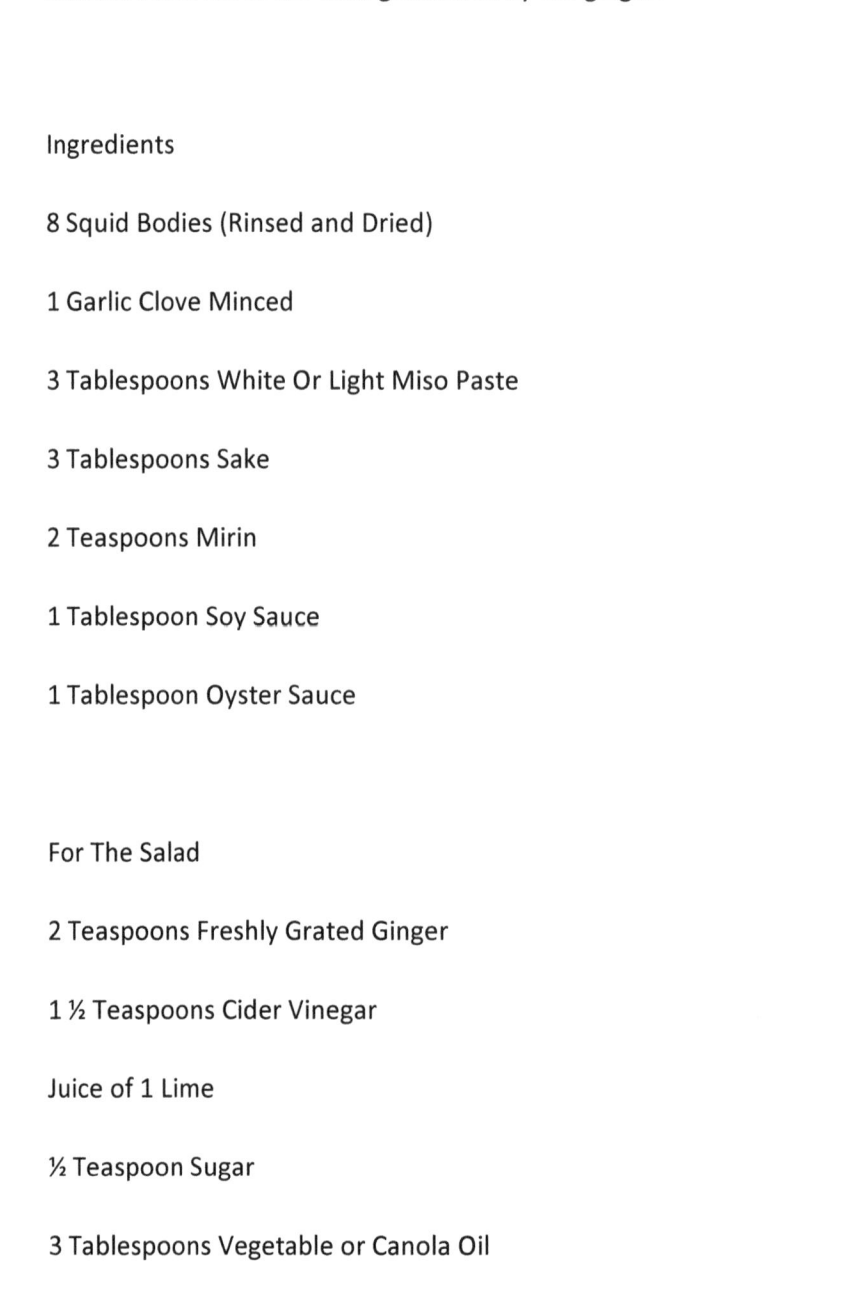

Ingredients

8 Squid Bodies (Rinsed and Dried)

1 Garlic Clove Minced

3 Tablespoons White Or Light Miso Paste

3 Tablespoons Sake

2 Teaspoons Mirin

1 Tablespoon Soy Sauce

1 Tablespoon Oyster Sauce

For The Salad

2 Teaspoons Freshly Grated Ginger

1 ½ Teaspoons Cider Vinegar

Juice of 1 Lime

½ Teaspoon Sugar

3 Tablespoons Vegetable or Canola Oil

5 Stalks of Celery Halved Lengthways then Sliced Diagonally into 2 ½ inch pieces

1 Tart Apple (Granny Smith is Ideal) Peeled then Cut Into Matchstick Size Pieces

2 Green Onions Halved Lengthways Then Slice Into 2 ½ inch Matchsticks (Use the white and pale green parts only)

110grams Sunflower Sprouts

1 Serrano Chili Halved Lengthways, Seeds Removed And Thinly Sliced Crosswise

1 Teaspoon Black Sesame Seeds

Coarse Salt to Taste

Instructions

1. In a saucepan mix together the garlic, white or light miso paste, sake, mirin, soy sauce and oyster sauce to make a marinade. You need to cook this sauce over a medium to high heat for around 3 minutes, making sure that you stir it continuously. After the 3 minutes have elapsed remove from heat and place in a bowl to cool slightly.

2. You now need to tenderize the squid to do this you need to pound both sides of it with a kitchen mallet a few times. Then cut along the seam of the squid with a sharp knife so you can open it up and lightly score the inside at ¼ inch intervals. After doing this add the squid to the marinade and leave it to stand for 20 minutes.

3. Whilst the squid is marinating in the sauce you can now make the dressing to go with the salad that you will serve with the grilled

squid. First of all you need to whisk together the ginger, lime juice, vinegar, sugar and salt and add the oil to it very slowly until the liquid becomes emulsified.

4. To cook the squid on the barbecue you need to make sure that it is preheated to a medium to high heat. When the barbecue is heated up you can now cook the squid. You will need to use something to put on top of the squid as it is cooking lining a skillet with aluminum foil and put something like bricks in it should help.

5. Before you place the squid on the grill sprinkle the scored sides of the squid with salt and then place them facing down on to the grill. It is a good idea to lightly oil the grill first before placing the squid on it to prevent them from sticking.

Once you have placed the squid on the grill place the weighted skillet on top and let them cook for about 1 ½ minutes. Once the squid is cooked remove and cut into ¾ inch pieces.

6. To finish off take the apple, celery, green onions, sprouts and chilli into a bowl and pour over 3 tablespoons of the dressing made earlier. Toss the ingredients so that they are all coated in the dressing then place some on to a clean plate with some of the squid on top before then sprinkling over this some sesame seeds.

RECIPE 38 – MONKFISH & PRAWN KEBABS WITH TOMATO SALSA

These kebabs taste really wonderful when served with a Mexican style tomato sauce.

Samantha Michaels

Ingredients

700grams Monkfish Tail

100grams about 4 Large Raw Tiger Prawns or 8 to 12 Smaller Ones

1 Garlic Clove Crushed

1 Teaspoon Ginger Puree or Freshly Grated Ginger

1 Green Chilli (Deseeded and Finely Chopped)

1 Tablespoon Sunflower or Ground Nut Oil

Salt and Freshly Ground Black Pepper To Taste

Salsa

500grams Plum Tomatoes

2 Teaspoons Coriander Seeds

1 Green Chilli (Deseeded and Finely Chopped)

1 Garlic Clove Crushed

1 Stalk Lemongrass (Outer Leaves Removed Then Finely Sliced)

Juice of 1 Lime

Wedges of Lime To Serve

With Dish

Instructions

1. Rinse the monkfish in cold water and then pat dry with paper towels. Remove any grey membrane and then cut the flesh away from the backbone cartilage so you have two long pieces. Then cut each piece into equal size chunks. You should aim to get between 8 and 12 chunks from each piece.

2. Next you need to peel the prawns if you can leave the tails on and just remove the legs and heads. Now run a sharp knife along the back of each prawn and pull out the dark thread running through him or her. Then rinse them in cold water then pat dry and put to one side for use later as with the monkfish.

NB: It would be a good idea to put the monkfish and prawns in the refrigerator until needed.

3. Now you are ready to start making the marinade for the kebabs. To do this mix the garlic, chilli, ginger and oil in a bowl and then to this add the monkfish and prawns and mix all ingredients together well. Now cover the top of the bowl with cling film and place in the refrigerator for 1 hour. Whilst the fish and prawns are marinating take your wooden skewers and place them in some water to soak.

4. Whilst the monkfish and prawns are marinating you can begin making the salsa. First off you need to cover the tomatoes with boiling water and then leave them like this for one minute. After a minute has passed remove the tomatoes from the water and peel away the skin and cut in half so that you can remove the seeds. Now cut each half of the tomato into chunky puree. Unfortunately you will have to do this by hand rather than using a food processor.

5. Now place the chunks of tomato into a bowl and into this mix the chilli, garlic, lime juice and lemongrass. Then add a little salt and pepper to taste. Cover the bowl over and place in the refrigerator ready for when you want to serve the kebabs.

6. To cook the kebabs you need to place them on the barbecue grill on a medium to high heat and cook each one for between 3 to 4 minutes on both sides. You can tell when the kebabs are ready, as the prawns will have turned a pink color and feel much firmer. You should have threaded onto each skewer chunks of monkfish and 1, 2 or 3 prawns (dependent on their size).

Recipe 39 – Skewered Swordfish With Charred Courgettes

Swordfish is ideally suited to being cooked on skewers because the flesh is so firm. Serve this particular dish with some warm focaccia bread.

Ingredients

500grams Swordfish Steaks Cut Into 2cm Chunks

3 Lemons

3 Tablespoon Olive Oil

1 Garlic Clove Crushed

15grams Fresh Basil Chopped

500grams Small Courgettes Trimmed

Barbecue Cookbook

Instructions

1. Whilst four long wooden skewers are soaking in water you need to cut the swordfish up into 2cm chunks. To do this you first need to cut away the skin. As the skin is quite thick you need to use a very sharp knife.

2. In a bowl grate the zest from one of the lemons and add to this the juice of it along with the olive oil and garlic and then add to it the finely chopped up basil leaves then mix well together. As for the other two lemons you now need to cut these into 8 wedges.

3. Next cut the courgettes in half lengthways and then score the white flesh with the tip of a sharp knife so a criss cross pattern is formed on them. Then lightly brush with some of the marinade you have just made and set to one side for cooking on the barbecue later.

4. Now into the marinade you need to put the chunks of swordfish and mix well together before then placing to one side for them to marinate in the sauce for between 5 and 10 minutes. Whilst the swordfish is marinating in the sauce now is the time to turn on or light your barbecue.

5. As soon as the marinating time has elapsed you are now ready to make up the kebabs on to each skewer thread chunks of swordfish along with the lemon wedges in an alternate pattern. Then sprinkle both the kebabs and courgettes with some coarsely ground black pepper and place all items on to the barbecue grill, which has been lightly oiled.

6. Cook both the kebabs and courgettes for between 10 and 15 minutes, making sure that you turn the kebabs over occasionally to ensure that the fish is cooked right through. The same also goes for the courgettes. It is important that whilst the kebabs are cooking that you also baste them regularly with any marinade you have left

over. Once the kebabs and courgettes are cooked serve to guests on clean plates along with the warm focaccia bread.

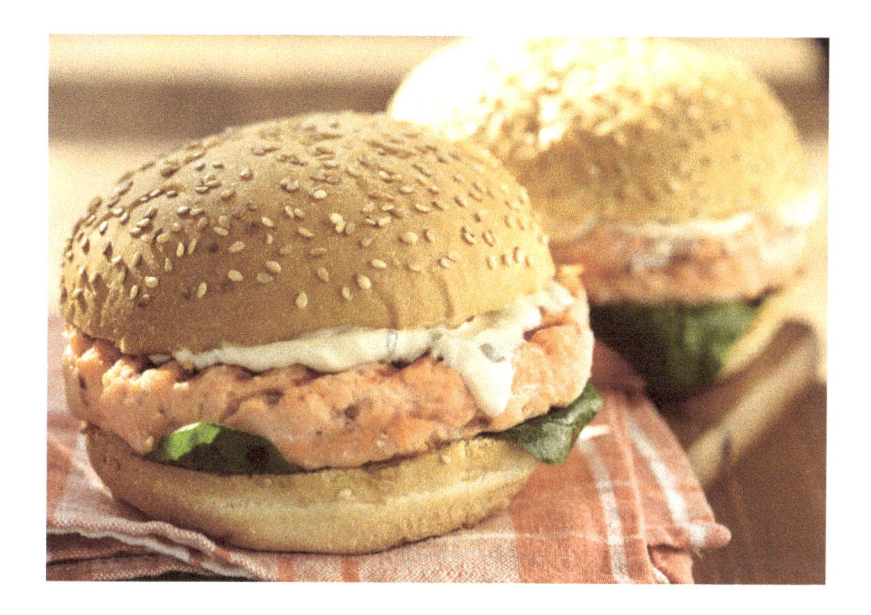

RECIPE 40 – ROSEMARY SALMON BURGERS

You may find it hard to believe but this burgers hold up extremely well when cooked on a barbecue. If you can use a good fillet of wild salmon to make the burgers from. Once cooked serve the burgers in a roll with some lettuce and tomato and a mustard and horseradish sauce.

Ingredients

1Kg King Salmon Fillet (Skinned and Bones Removed)

100grams Dried Breadcrumbs

80grams Minced Red Onion

1 Tablespoon Dijon Mustard

2 Teaspoons Horseradish (Freshly Grated If Possible)

2 Eggs (That Have Been Lightly Beaten)

1 Tablespoon Fresh Rosemary Minced

½ Teaspoon Salt

½ Teaspoon Freshly Ground Black Pepper

2 Tablespoons Olive Oil

Instructions

1. You need to cut the salmon into strips crossways and then chopping these up until the fish has become well minced. As you do chop the fish up look out for any bones and remove these.

2. Now into a large bowl place the minced salmon, breadcrumbs, red onion, mustard, horseradish and eggs. Then season this mixture with the salt and pepper and rosemary and combine them all together. Now place the mixture in the refrigerator to chill for at least 30 minutes. Whilst the salmon mixture is chilling you should now get your barbecue going and place the grill which you will have oiled just before you start cooking around 4 to 6 inches above the heat source. This is because you will be cooking the burgers on a medium to high heat.

3. After removing the salmon mixture from the refrigerator form it into 8 burger patter and then lightly coat each one with some olive oil. Then place each patty on the barbecue and cook for between 4 and 5 minutes on each side. As soon as the burgers are cooked

serve on a bun with lettuce and tomato and pot of mustard and horseradish beside them.

RECIPE 41 – FAST FISH KEBABS

Even though this recipe allows you to cook the fish quickly you will need to allow plenty of time for the fish to marinate. At least 2 hours should be sufficient time. If you can use any fish with firm flesh to make your kebabs from. Swordfish is ideal.

Ingredients

750grams Firm Fish Fillets

2 Tablespoons Olive Oil

1 Garlic Clove Finely Chopped

1 Tablespoon Fresh Coriander Chopped

1 Teaspoon Ground Cumin

1 Teaspoon Lemon Juice (Fresh If Possible)

Salt and Freshly Ground Black Pepper To Taste

Instructions

1. In a bowl combine together the olive oil, garlic, coriander, cumin, lemon juice, salt and pepper, then place to one side, as this is the marinade for the fish.

2. Now take the fish fillets and cut these in to 3cm size cubes and combine with the sauce you made earlier. Now place the covered bowl into a refrigerator for several hours. Whilst the fish is marinating make sure that you stir it occasionally.

3. Just before you are about to start threading the fish cubes on to wooden skewers that have been soaking in water for at least 30 minutes you should get the barbecue going.

4. It is important that before you thread the cubes of fish on to the skewers you drain them well first and also make sure that the grill on the barbecue has been oiled. Now place the skewers on the barbecue and cook each kebab for between 6 and 8 minutes turning them occasionally and also basting them with any leftover marinade. The fish is cooked through when the flesh has turned opaque and the exterior is a light brown color.

Once the kebabs are cooked serve them with a crisp green salad and some lemon wedges.

RECIPE 42 – BARBECUED HALIBUT STEAKS

Although this is a very simple fish dish for cooking on the barbecue it tastes extremely delicious.

Ingredients

450grams Halibut Steak

30grams Butter

2 Tablespoons Dark Brown Soft Sugar

Samantha Michaels

1 Tablespoon Lemon Juice

2 Teaspoons Soy Sauce

½ Teaspoon Freshly Ground Black Pepper

Instructions

1. Place in a small saucepan over a medium heat the butter, sugar, garlic, lemon juice, soy sauce and pepper. Stir this mixture occasionally and remove from heat as soon as all the sugar has dissolved.

2. Lightly oil your preheated barbecue with some oil and just before you place the halibut steaks on to it lightly brush each side with the sauce you made earlier. Cook each side of the fish for about 5 minutes or until the flesh of the fish can be flaked easily with a fork. Whilst the fish is cooking make sure that you keep basting with the sauce.

3. Once the fish is cooked serve to your guests on a plate with some warm new potatoes and a crisp green salad. Otherwise you may want to consider serving the fish with some rice.

Chapter 6 - Shellfish Recipes

Recipe 1 – Grilled King Crab Legs

Of all the recipes we provide in this book this really is the simplest among them.

Ingredients

450grams King Crab Legs per Person

2 Tablespoons Olive Oil

2 Tablespoons Melted Butter

Instructions

1. Preheat the barbecue and place the grill around 6 inches above the heat source as the crabs legs will need to be cooked on a medium heat. Whilst the barbecue is heating up in a bowl mix together the olive oil and butter and then brush this over the crab legs.

2. Now place the crab legs on the grill, which you may want to lightly oil as well and close the lid on your barbecue. Now let the legs cook on the barbecue for between 4 and 5 minutes making sure that halfway through you turn them over.

3. Once the crab legs are cooked remove from the barbecue and serve them with some fresh crusty bread along with a cocktail or garlic butter sauce. To make the garlic butter sauce in a sauce pan place 50grams of melted butter with 1 tablespoon of freshly

chopped garlic and heat gently. Doing this will then allow the flavor of the garlic to become infused in the butter.

RECIPE 2 – SPICY SHRIMP SKEWERS

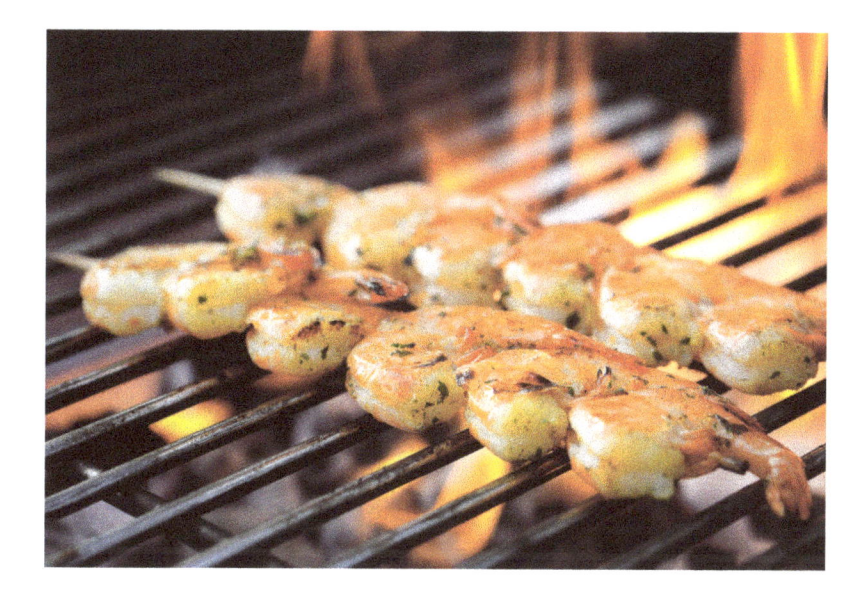

This is the perfect recipe to serve at any barbecue in the summer. The perfect accompaniment to this dish is seasoned rice along with frozen margaritas.

Ingredients

900grams Large Shrimps (Peeled and Deveined)

80ml Fresh Lime Juice

80ml Honey

1 Teaspoon Soy Sauce

Barbecue Cookbook

1 Teaspoon Vegetable Oil

2 Tablespoons Jamaican Jerk Seasoning

3 Dashes Hot Pepper Sauce

Salt and Freshly Ground Black Pepper to Taste

12 Wooden Skewers That Have Been Soaked In Water for 1 Hour

Instructions

1. In a bowl combine together the lime juice, honey, soy sauce and oil. Then to this add the Jamaican jerk seasoning, hot pepper sauce, salt and pepper.

2. Now add to the sauce you have just made the shrimps make sure that you mix everything well together so that the shrimps are completely coated in the sauce. Cover the bowl and place in the refrigerator and leave there for one hour to allow the shrimps to marinate in the sauce. This is the time when the skewers should have been placed in the water to soak.

3. About 30 minutes before the shrimps are due to come out the refrigerator you should now get your barbecue going. The shrimps will need to be cooked on a medium to high heat so place the grill of the barbecue about 4 to 6 inches above the heat source.

4. After removing the shrimps from the refrigerator now remove the skewers from the water, then pat them dry before then spraying or brushing with some nonstick cooking spray or oil. Now thread on to each skewer the shrimps until all 12 skewers have been used and place on the grill and cook each kebab for 5 minutes on each side or until the shrimps have turned pink in color.

Once the shrimps are cooked place on clean plates and serve with the seasoned rice and frozen margaritas.

RECIPE 3 – GRILLED OYSTERS

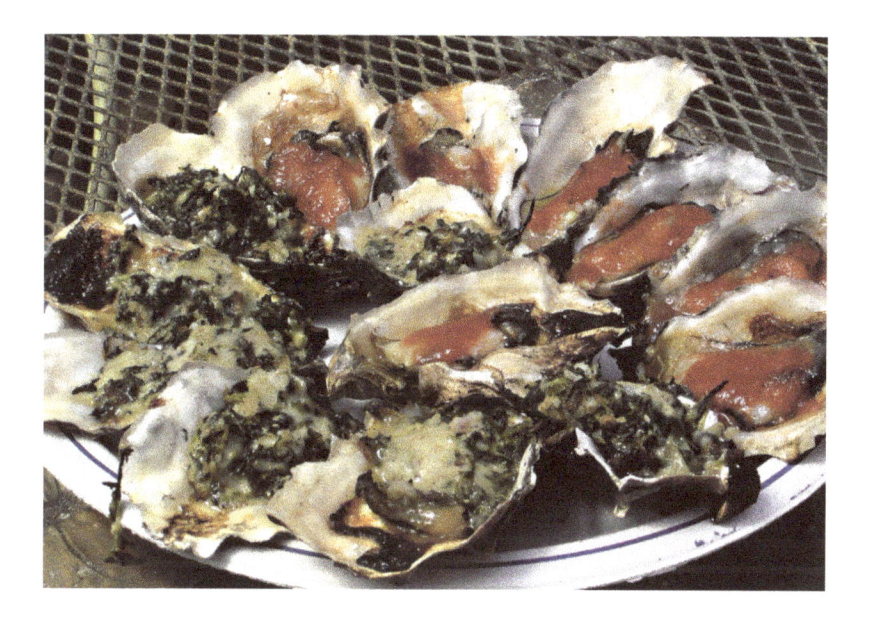

It is important that you make sure that you clean the oysters very well. However you may find that they have already been cleaned well by your fishmonger and so will only need a light scrubbing and rinsing. Whilst you are cleaning the oysters make sure that they are tightly closed. If they aren't or you find that they are easy to open through them away as these aren't fresh or healthy. After cleaning the oysters keep them cold by placing them in a bowl with a bag ice on top.

Ingredients

12 to 18 Oysters for Each Person

Melted Butter

Hot Sauce

Worcestershire Sauce

Instructions

1. Once the barbecue has heated up place the oysters on to the grill on a medium to high heat. If you want to prevent any flare ups whilst the oysters are cooking as juices drip out of them then cover the grill with some aluminum foil first.

2. After placing the oysters on the grill close the lid of the barbecue and let them cook. It is important that you keep a close eye on the oysters as they are cooking. So check them every 3 to 4 minutes. Once you notice the shells starting to open then remove them from the grill.

3. After removing the oysters from the grill open the shells and then loosen the meat and place on a plate so your guests can then help themselves. Beside the plate of oysters put some bowls with the melted butter, hot sauce and Worcestershire sauce in them and which the guests can then spoon on top of the oysters if they wish. Then simply pop in the mouth and enjoy.

RECIPE 4 – THAI SPICED PRAWNS

If you are looking for a barbecued prawn recipe that comes with a little kick then this is the one for you.

Samantha Michaels

Ingredients

450grams Medium Size Prawns (Peeled and Deveined)

3 Tablespoons Fresh Lemon Juice

1 Tablespoon Soy Sauce

1 Tablespoon Dijon Mustard

2 Garlic Cloves Minced

1 Tablespoon Brown Sugar

2 Teaspoons Curry Paste

Instructions

1. In either a resealable plastic bag or a shallow baking dish mix together the lemon juice, soy sauce, mustard, garlic, sugar and curry paste. Then add the prawns and mix all these ingredients together thoroughly. Now seal up the bag or cover the dish with some cling film and place in the refrigerator to marinate for 1 hour.

2. Next heat up the barbecue and place the grill down low as you will be cooking these prawns on a high heat. Once the barbecue is ready lightly oil the grill and place the prawns that have been threaded onto skewers and cook on each side for 3 minutes each. If you want to make turning them over easier place the kebabs inside a fish basket. You will know when the prawns are ready, as they will turn a pink opaque color.

3. As for the remaining sauce, which you marinated the prawns in initially, transfer this to a small saucepan and heat up until it starts to boil. Allow it to boil for a few minutes before then transferring

to a bowl which your guests can then dip the kebabs in and which you have also used to baste the prawns in whilst cooking.

RECIPE 5 – GARLIC GRILLED SHRIMPS

You can serve these shrimps either with pasta or salad or as fajitas to your guests.

Ingredients

450grams Large Size Shrimps (Peeled and Deveined)

4 Garlic Cloves

Salt to Taste

30ml Olive Oil

¼ Teaspoon Freshly Ground Black Pepper to Taste

Instructions

1. Start the barbecue up and lightly oil the grill.

2. Now take the four garlic cloves and chop them up then sprinkle with some salt and using the back of a large knife smash the garlic up until it forms a paste. Then place the garlic with some olive oil in a frying pan (skillet) and cook over a medium to low heat until the garlic starts to turn brown. This should take around 5 minutes then once the garlic has turned brown remove from heat.

3. Next you take the shrimps and thread them onto wooden skewers and sprinkle over them some salt and pepper to season. Then brush one side of the shrimps with the garlic and olive oil mixture you made earlier and place this side down on to the barbecue.

4. Cook the shrimps until they start to turn pink in color and they begin to curl. This should take around 4 minutes and then turn them over. But before placing back down on the barbecue brush with more of the garlic oil and then cook for a further 4 minutes until the flesh has turned opaque and the shrimps are pink all over.

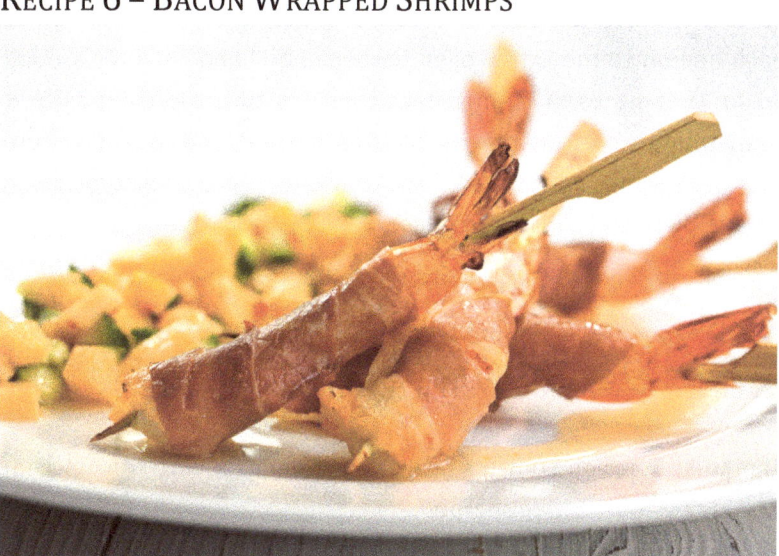

RECIPE 6 – BACON WRAPPED SHRIMPS

Can either be served as an appetizer to your guests as they arrive or as a starter.

Ingredients

16 Large Shrimps (Peeled and Deveined)

8 Slices of Bacon

Barbecue Seasoning to Taste

Instructions

1. Preheat the barbecue and place the grill about 4 to 6 inches above the heat.

2. Take each shrimp and wrap them in half of each slice of bacon and then secure with a toothpick or thread two of them on to a wooden skewer that has been soaking in water for 30 minutes.

3. Now sprinkle some of the seasoning over them and then place each one on to the lightly oiled barbecue grill and cook for around 10 to 15 minutes. It is important that you turn the shrimps over frequently to prevent the bacon from burning and also to ensure that the shrimps are cooked through evenly. Once cooked place on a clean plate and allow your guests to help themselves.

Recipe 7 – Scallops With A Herb & Pecan Crust

The crust that you coat the scallops with adds a very fresh accent to this delicious tasting seafood.

Ingredients

450grams Scallops (About 12 to 15 Scallops)

64grams Toasted Pecan Pieces

43grams Fresh Oregano Leaves

Samantha Michaels

32grams Fresh Thyme Leaves

3 Garlic Cloves Chopped

2 Teaspoons Chicken Flavored Bouillon Granules

1 Teaspoon Freshly Shredded Lemon Peel

¼ Teaspoon Freshly Ground Black Pepper

3 Tablespoons Olive Oil

Instructions

1. In a food processor place the pecan pieces, oregano, thyme, garlic, bouillon granules, lemon peel and black pepper. Turn machine on until they form a paste then very slowly and gradually add the olive oil.

2. Once you have formed a paste now rub it onto the scallops and then thread three of each on to a skewer. If you are using wooden ones remember to soak in water for at least 30 minutes to prevent them from burning when on the barbecue.

3. Once the scallops are ready on the skewers place on the preheated barbecue over a medium heat so set the grill about 6 inches above the heat source and cook them for between 5 and 8 minutes. The best way of knowing when the scallops are ready to serve is to see if they have turned opaque in color.

4. As soon as the scallops are cooked serve to your guests on clean plates with some crusty bread and a crisp green salad that has been drizzled with lemon juice and olive oil.

Recipe 8 – Grilled Oysters With Fennel Butter

This particular recipe cannot only be served as a main dish to your guests but as an accompaniment to others.

Ingredients

24 Fresh Live Unopened Medium Size Oysters

1 Teaspoon Grounded Fennel Seed

226grams Softened Butter

1 Tablespoon Minced Shallots

1 Tablespoon Chopped Fennel Greens

1 Teaspoon Freshly Ground Black Pepper

½ Teaspoon Salt

Instructions

1. Get the barbecue going so and place the grill down low as possible as you will be cooking the oysters on a very high heat.

2. In a bowl mix together the butter, fennel seeds, shallots, fennel greens, pepper and salt. Then put to one side for use later. If you want place in the refrigerator to keep the butter from melting completely and remove about 10 minutes before needed.

3. Place the oysters on the grill of the barbecue and close the lid and leave it closed for between 3 and 5 minutes or until you start to hear them hiss or they start to open.

4. Take an oyster knife and pry each one of the oysters open at the hinge and loosen the oyster inside. Discard the flat part of the shell and then top each of the open oysters with ½ teaspoon of the butter you made earlier and then return them back to the barbecue once more. Then cook them once more until the butter has melted and is hot.

Recipe 9 – Grilled Crab

Most people don't think that cooking things such as crabs on a barbecue is a good idea. But it is because the direct heat and flavor help to make this one of the best ways of cooking most types of shellfish today.

Ingredients

2 Large Live Crabs

60ml White Wine Vinegar

2 ½ Teaspoons Sugar

2 Tablespoons Olive Oil

1 Tablespoon Freshly Minced Ginger

1 Jalapeno Chili Seeds Removed Then Minced

1 Tablespoon Minced Cilantro

1 Medium Tomato Chopped

Instructions

1. In a bowl mix together the chopped tomato, vinegar, oil, ginger, chili, garlic and cilantro. Then place to one side for use later.

2. Now into a large pot of boiling water place the crabs one at the time head first. Reduce the heat and allow the crabs to sit in simmering water for 5 minutes before then removing. If however you find the thought of cooking live crabs a little too much then you can use frozen ones instead. Of course you need to allow them sufficient time to thaw out before you can start cooking with them.

3. After removing the crabs from the water turn over and pull the triangular tab from the belly and lift of the shell. Remove the entrails and gills from the crab before then washing and draining. Now place on the barbecue that you have preheated and close the lid. But before closing the lid brush with the mixture you made earlier and do this regularly throughout the time the crabs are grilling on the barbecue.

4. About halfway through the cooking time (around about 5minutes) you need to turn the crabs over and repeat the same process again for a further 5 minutes or until the meat in the legs of the crabs has turned opaque.

5. Now place the crabs on to a plate to serve them but before you do serve spoon over any remaining sauce you have that you used to baste the crabs in when cooking. If you wish you can put the meat back in the shells before serving.

Recipe 10 – Sesame Scallops

This marinade helps to enhance the flavor of the scallops even further. Best served either on a bed of noodles, rice or with some grilled vegetables.

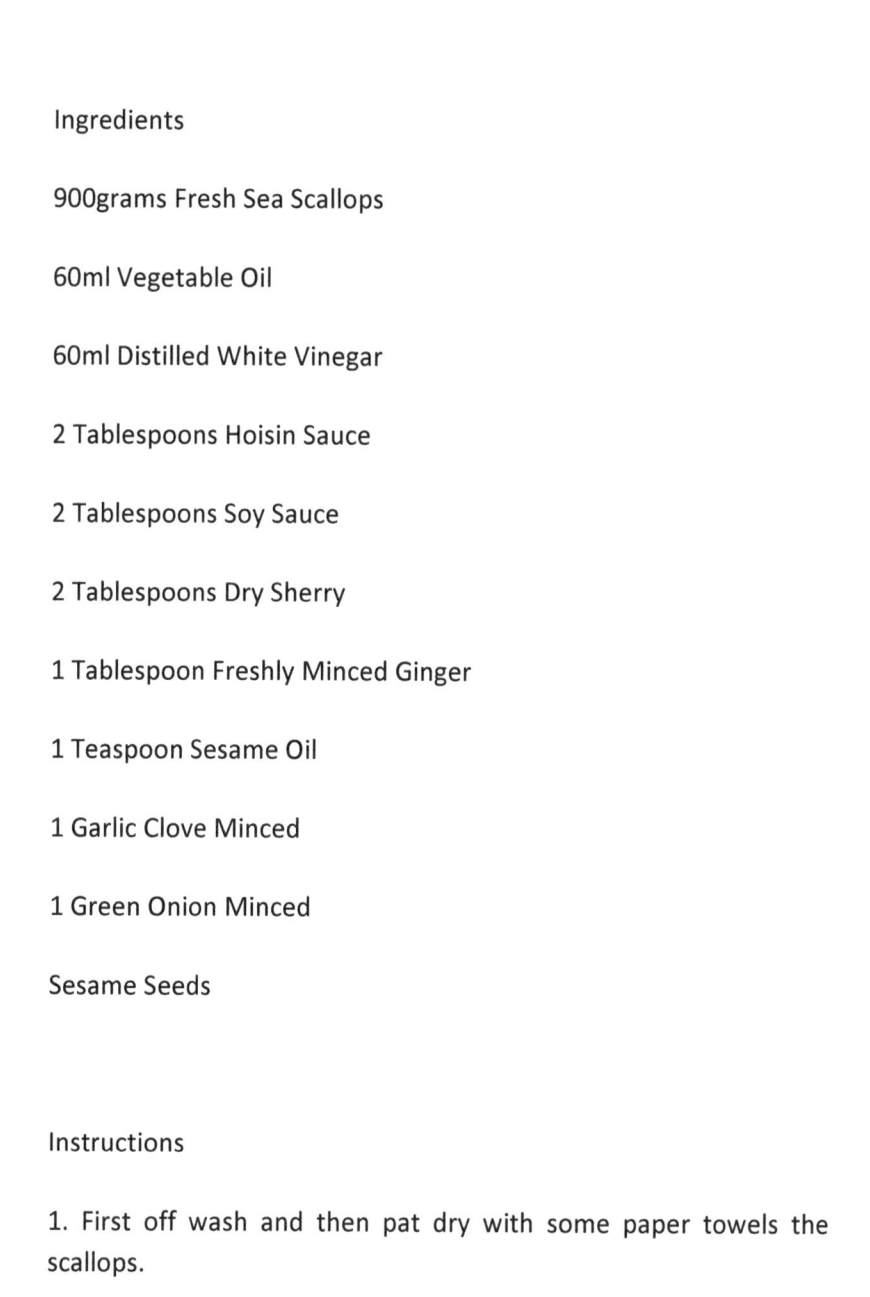

Ingredients

900grams Fresh Sea Scallops

60ml Vegetable Oil

60ml Distilled White Vinegar

2 Tablespoons Hoisin Sauce

2 Tablespoons Soy Sauce

2 Tablespoons Dry Sherry

1 Tablespoon Freshly Minced Ginger

1 Teaspoon Sesame Oil

1 Garlic Clove Minced

1 Green Onion Minced

Sesame Seeds

Instructions

1. First off wash and then pat dry with some paper towels the scallops.

2. Now into a bowl mix together the oil, vinegar, hoisin and soy sauce, dry sherry, ginger, sesame oil, garlic and onion. Then pour this mixture into a resealable bag and then add to these the scallops. Turn the bag over several times to ensure that all the scallops are covered in the marinade and place in the refrigerator overnight.

3. Whilst the barbecue is heating up you can now remove the scallops from the refrigerator and thread them on to skewers ready for cooking. Once placed on the skewers then sprinkle over some of the sesame seeds and cook over a medium heat (so place the grill about 4 to 6 inches above the heat source) and cook for 6 to 8 minutes. You will know the scallops are ready to eat when they have turned opaque.

Recipe 11 – Margarita Shrimps

If you wish you can marinate the shrimps in this sauce for up to 3 hours. Plus you can increase or reduce the amount of red pepper included in this dish dependent on how hot you like your food to be.

Ingredients

450grams Shrimps (Peeled and Deveined)

2 Garlic Cloves Minced

2 Tablespoons Fresh Lime Juice

3 Tablespoons Olive Oil

2 Teaspoons Tequila

Samantha Michaels

3 Tablespoons Freshly Chopped Cilantro

¼ Teaspoon Ground Red Pepper

¼ Teaspoon Salt

Instructions

1. In a bowl place the lime juice, olive oil, tequila, garlic, cilantro, pepper and salt and combine well together before then adding the shrimps. Toss the mixture about lightly to ensure that the shrimps are covered in the sauce then cover the bowl and place in the refrigerator for between 30 minutes and 3 hours to marinate.

2. Turn on or light the barbecue about 30 minutes prior to when you want to start cooking the shrimps. You need to place the grill down low in the barbecue, as you will be cooking these on a high heat for a very short space of time.

3. Whilst the barbecue is heating up take the shrimps out of the fridge and thread them on to either metal or wooden skewers. Put about 3 or 4 on each skewer and place to one side. If there is any marinade left over in the bowl discard this.

4. Before you place the shrimps on to the barbecue grill lightly oil it first to prevent the shrimps from sticking to it. Now cook the shrimps for between 2 and 3 minutes on each side or until they have turned pink. Then serve.

Barbecue Cookbook

RECIPE 12 – BAJA STYLE GRILLED ROCK LOBSTER TAILS

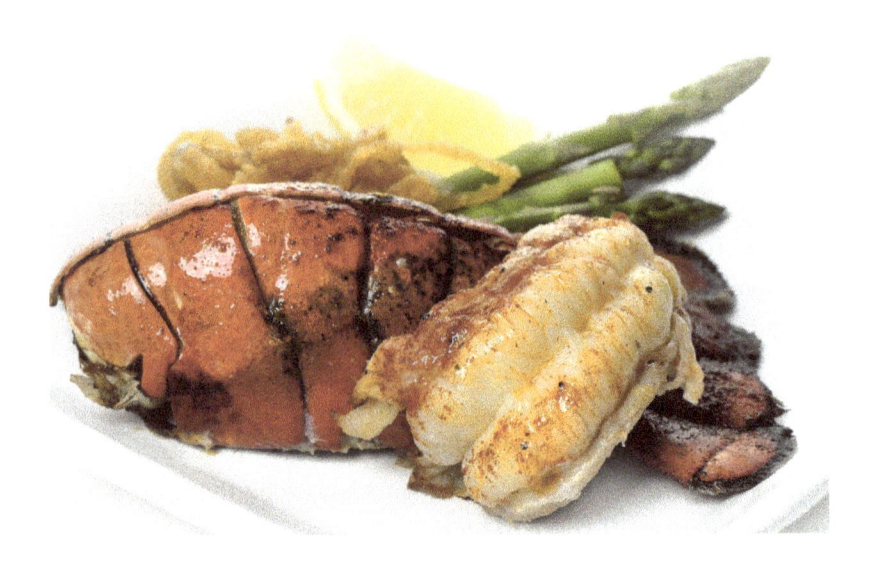

This very simple citrus sauce complements the richness of the lobster tails very well. Best served with warm tortillas and lightly grilled green onions. To cut the tails in half you should use either kitchen shears or a cleaver. If you want to give this dish a more authentic Mexican flavor then douse the tails in a hot Mexican sauce like Cholula.

Ingredients

6 x 226gram Rock or Spiny Lobster Tails

12 Green Onions

Sauce

1 Tablespoon Grated Orange Rind

2 Tablespoons Freshly Squeezed Orange Juice

1 Tablespoon Freshly Squeezed Lemon Juice

1 Tablespoon Olive Oil

½ Teaspoon Dried Oregano

¼ Teaspoon Salt

Dash of Hot Sauce (Such as Cholula)

1 Garlic Clove Minced

2 Tablespoons Melted Butter

Instructions

1. Get the barbecue going so it is ready in time for cooking to begin.

2. Now you need to start preparing the lobster. To do this cut each lobster tail in half lengthwise and then coat each one along with the onions with some cooking spray.

3. Next place the tails on to the grill of the barbecue cut side facing downwards and after you have oiled the grill lightly. Grill the tails for 3 minutes and then turn them over. Now grill them for a further five minutes.

4. About 2 minutes after turning over the tails now place the green onions on the grill to cook. These will require about 3 minutes and should be turned over at least once during this cooking time. Remove from barbecue once they have become tender.

Barbecue Cookbook

5. To make the sauce which you will serve with the lobster tails in to a bowl place the orange rind, orange juice, lime juice, olive oil, oregano, salt, hot sauce and garlic and whisk well. Then very gradually add to this mixture the melted butter making sure that you whisk the ingredients continuously then drizzle it over the cut side of the tails.

6. Transfer to a clean plate and serve along side them some warm tortillas and some lime wedges.

Recipe 13 – Grilled Prawns With Spicy Peanut Lime Vinaigrette

Not only does this Thai inspired sauce go very well with prawns but you may also want to try it with chicken, lamb or pork.

Ingredients

900grams (16-20) Extra Large Shrimps (Peeled and Deveined But Tails Left On)

32grams Minced Lemon Grass (White Part Only)

32grams Fresh Minced Ginger Root

2 Tablespoons Minced Garlic

¼ Tablespoon Freshly Chopped Cilantro

1 Thai or Serrano Chili Minced

180ml Peanut or Canola Oil

Vinaigrette

60ml Lime Juice

60ml Rice Wine Vinegar

120ml Japanese Sweet Wine (Mirin)

2 Tablespoons Dark Soy Sauce

2 Tablespoons Cold Water

3 Tablespoons Grated Lime Zest

1 Tablespoon Freshly Minced Ginger Root

2 Teaspoons Fish Sauce

2 Fresh Thai or Serrano Chilli's (Seeds Removed)

2 Teaspoons Minced Garlic

113grams Unsalted Smooth Peanut Butter

30ml Peanut Oil

2 Tablespoons Freshly Chopped Mint

1 Tablespoon Freshly Chopped Cilantro

57grams Chopped Unsalted Roasted Peanuts

Salt to Taste

Instructions

1. In a bowl (large) combine together the ginger, lemon grass, garlic, cilantro, chili and oil. Then add the shrimps and let them marinate in the sauce made for 20 to 30 minutes at room temperature.

2. Whilst the shrimps are marinating in the sauce you can now start heating up the barbecue placing the grill about 6 inches above the heat source. This will then enable you to cook the shrimps that you will thread on to skewers on a medium to high heat.

3. Now into a food processor place the lime juice, rice vinegar, mirin, soy sauce and water and blend. Then add to this the lime zest, ginger, fish sauce, chilies, garlic and peanut butter and process until the mixture becomes smooth. Whilst these ingredients are combining together slowly pour in the peanut oil until the mixture looks smooth and creamy.

Pour this mixture into a bowl and then stir into it the mint, cilantro and chopped peanuts. Add some salt if needed.

4. To cook the shrimps remove them from the marinade, shaking off any excess and thread them on to skewers then cook them on either side for about 2 minutes or until they have turned pink and firm. Once cooked serve on a plate immediately with the sauce beside them.

RECIPE 14 – SCALLOPS & CHERRY TOMATO KEBABS

The applying of fresh lemon juice and Dijon mustard to these scallops and tomato kebabs helps to give them a much spicier and tarter flavor.

Samantha Michaels

Ingredients

16 Large Sea Scallops

24 Cherry Tomatoes

1 Lemon

2 Tablespoons Olive Oil

2 Tablespoons Dijon Mustard

1/8 Teaspoon Salt

Instructions

1. Start preparing the barbecue for cooking this dish on a medium heat. This means putting the grill of the barbecue about 6 inches above the main heat source. Also place the wooden skewers in some water.

2. Whilst the barbecue is heating up you can now prepare the sauce for the kebabs. In a bowl place 1 tablespoon of lemon juice along with ½ teaspoon of its peel. To this then add the olive oil, Dijon mustard and salt and mix well together. Then put to one side ready for use later.

3. Now on to each of the wooden skewers you need to thread 3 tomatoes and 2 scallops alternately. You should start and finish with the tomatoes.

4. Next brush the kebabs you have just made with some of the sauce you made earlier and place on the barbecue to cook. Each kebab will need to cook for between 7 and 9 minutes and should be turned over several times. After this time has elapsed brush the kebabs with the remainder of the sauce and then cook for another

5 minutes or more remembering to turn them over frequently. The kebabs will be ready to consume when the scallops have turned opaque right through.

5. Once the kebabs are cooked served to your guests immediately with a little green salad and some crusty bread.

RECIPE 15 – GRILLED LOBSTER WITH LIME BAY BUTTER

This is quite an easy dish to do. However before the lobsters are placed on the barbecue they need to be parboiled first.

Ingredients

3 x 680grams Fresh Lobsters

113grams Butter

60ml Fresh Lime Juice

½ Teaspoon Crushed Bay Leaf

¼ Teaspoon Freshly Ground Black Pepper

¼ Teaspoon Salt

Instructions

1. To parboil the lobsters you need to bring around 3 inches of water to boil in an 8 quart saucepan. Once the water begins boiling add the lobsters, then cover the pan and cook for 10 minutes. Once the 10 minutes has elapsed remove the lobsters from the pan and leave them to one side to cool.

2. Whilst the barbecue is heating up in another saucepan place the butter, lime juice, bay leaf, salt and pepper and cook for 10 minutes over a low heat. Then put to one side to use later on.

3. By now the lobsters should have cooled down sufficiently to enable you to cut them in half lengthwise and brush them with the butter mixture you have just made.

4. After brushing the cut side of the lobster with the butter mixture you place them cut side down onto the grill of the barbecue which you have placed about 4 inches above the heat source and cook them for 5 minutes.

5. Now turn the lobsters over carefully brushing them with some more of the butter mixture and continuing cooking them on the barbecue until the meat is cooked through. This should take about another 5 minutes.

6. As soon as the meat is cooked through remove the lobsters from the barbecue place on a clean plate and garnish them with lime wedges and bay leaves if you want. Each of your guests should be given ½ lobster each.

RECIPE 16 – GRILLED PRAWNS & GARLIC CHILI SAUCE

The sauce you use with this particular recipe helps to enhance the sweetness of the prawns even further. Don't be surprised if you guests won't to know the secret to this great tasting dish.

Ingredients

450grams Jumbo Size Prawns (Devein Them)

2 Tablespoons Cooking Oil

2 Tablespoons Minced Garlic

2 Tablespoons Thinly Sliced Lemon Grass

5 Fresh Thai Chilli's Thinly Sliced

1 Shallot Thinly Sliced

2 Kaffir Lime Leaves

1 Tablespoon Fish Sauce

Juice Of 1 Lime

1 Tablespoon Thai Roasted Chilli Paste

1 Tablespoon Torn Fresh Mint Leaves

Instructions

1. Turn on or light your barbecue ready for cooking the prawns on. Placing the grill which has been lightly oiled about 6 inches above the heat sauce allowing you to cook the prawns on a medium heat.

2. Once the barbecue is heated up now place the prawns on to the grill and cook until the outside starts to turn pink and the meat inside no longer looks transparent. They will need to cook for between 5 and 10 minutes and should be turned over frequently. Whilst they are cooking you should now be making the sauce, which the prawns can then be dipped into.

3. To make the sauce heat some oil over a medium heat in a skillet and to this then add the garlic until it turns brown, which should take around 7 to 10 minutes. Now remove from the heat and to

the oil and garlic add the lemon grass, chilies, shallot, lime leaves, fish sauce, lime juice and chili paste. Toss to combine all these ingredients together then spoon some of them over the prawns, which you have removed from the barbecue and placed on a serving dish and the rest you pour into a bowl. Garnish with the freshly torn mint leaves.

Recipe 17 – Grilled New England Seafood

If you are looking for a recipe that doesn't take a great deal to prepare and won't leave you with too much mess afterwards this is one you should consider trying.

Ingredients

450grams Skinless Cod Fillet (Cut Into Four Equal Pieces)

225grams Frozen Uncooked Prawns (Peeled and Deveined and Thawed)

225grams Red New Potatoes (Skins Scrubbed then Thinly Sliced)

2 Ears of Corn Quartered

2 Tablespoons Butter (Room Temperature)

2 Tablespoons Finely Chopped Fresh Dill

1 Small Garlic Clove Minced

Coarse Salt and Freshly Ground Black Pepper To Taste

1 Lemon Thinly Sliced

Instructions

1. Start by getting your barbecue going and place the grill 6 inches above the heat source to allow the packets you are about to make to cook on a medium heat.

2. Whilst the barbecue is heating up in a bowl mix together the butter, dill, garlic, salt and pepper and place to one side for now.

3. Take four squares of aluminum foil measuring 14 inches square each. On to each of these four pieces of foil first place the thinly sliced potatoes before then placing on top of them a piece of the cod.

Next lay on some of the prawns and alongside the potatoes; cod and prawns place two pieces of the corn. Season each parcel with salt and pepper before adding a spoonful of the butter mixture on top. Then place on top of these two slices of the lemon.

4. Now bring up the sides of the foil and crimp the edges to seal the ingredients inside them tightly. Place each parcel on to the grill making sure that the potato is on the bottom and cook for about 12 to 14 minutes or until the fish is just cooked through and the potatoes are tender. You should make sure that you rotate not flip the parcels occasionally as this will help to ensure that everything inside is cooked properly.

5. Once the cooking time has passed remove the parcels from the heat and slit open the top of each one and transfer the contents to plates. If you want garnish the food with some more dill sprigs and serve some warm crusty rolls with them.

Recipe 18 – Honey Grilled Shrimps

Adding onions, peppers and mushrooms to this dish really helps to bring out even more of the beautiful flavors of the shrimps. You may also want to consider marinating the vegetables in the sauce along with the shrimps.

Ingredients

450grams Large Shrimps (Peeled and Deveined but with Tails still attached)

½ Teaspoon Garlic Powder

¼ Tablespoon Freshly Ground Black Pepper

80ml Worcestershire Sauce

2 Tablespoons Dry White Wine

2 Tablespoons Italian Style Salad Dressing

Honey Sauce

60ml Honey

57grams Melted Butter

2 Tablespoons Worcestershire Sauce

Instructions

1. Into a large bowl mix together the garlic powder, black pepper, Worcestershire sauce, dry white wine and the salad dressing. Then add the shrimp and toss them to coat them evenly in the marinade. Now cover the bowl over and place in the refrigerator to let the shrimp marinate in the sauce for 1 hour.

2. Start the barbecue up and place the grill, which needs to be lightly, oiled about 4 inches above the heat source to allow the shrimps to cook on a high heat. Remove the shrimps from the marinade and thread onto skewers. Pierce one through the head then the next one through the tail. Any marinade left over can now be discarded. Then set the shrimps to one side for a moment whilst you make the honey sauce.

3. To make the honey sauce in a small bowl mix together the honey melted butter and the other 2 tablespoons of Worcestershire sauce. This is what you will be basting the shrimps in as they cook.

4. Take the shrimps and place on the lightly oiled grill and cook for 2 to 3 minutes on each side, making sure you baste them occasionally with the honey sauce you have just made. You will know when the shrimps are ready to serve because the flesh will have turned opaque throughout. Serve to your guests immediately once cooked.

RECIPE 19 – SCALLOPS WRAPPED IN PROSCIUTTO

These will make a great starter to any barbecue and because they contain so few ingredients not only are they easy to prepare but also easy to cook.

Samantha Michaels

Ingredients

900grams (40) Medium Sized Scallops

450grams Paper Thin Slices Prosciutto

2 Lemons Halved

Freshly Ground Black Pepper

Extra Virgin Olive Oil (For Drizzling)

Instructions

1. Turn your gas barbecue on to high and allow to heat up whilst you are preparing the scallops for cooking. If you are using a charcoal barbecue you will know when it is hot enough when you can only hold your hand over it about 5 inches above the grill for 2 seconds.

2. Take one slice of the prosciutto and cut in half lengthwise then fold in half and wrap it around the sides of a scallop. You need to make sure that the ends of the prosciutto overlap and then thread it on to a skewer. Do the same for the other pieces of prosciutto and the scallops.

3. Next take the olive oil and drizzle it lightly over the scallops and then squeeze some lemon juice over them. Then season with the freshly ground black pepper. Then place on the barbecue to cook. Cook on each side for about 3 minutes or until you see the flesh of the scallops has turned opaque.

Remove from barbecue place on a clean plate with some lemon wedges and serve to your guests.

Barbecue Cookbook

RECIPE 20 – MAPLE ORANGE SHRIMP & SCALLOP KEBABS

Your guests will love the combination of the scallops and shrimps with the sweet citrus glaze. Make a wonderful entrée or starter to your barbecue. If you intend to serve as an entrée then place just one scallop and shrimp onto each skewer. If you intend to serve them as main course then serve with either steamed rice or seasonal vegetables or with a mixed green salad and light vinaigrette.

Ingredients

12 Jumbo Shrimps (Peeled and Deveined)

12 Large Sea Scallops

3 Tablespoons Vegetable Oil

½ Teaspoon Salt

½ Teaspoon Freshly Ground Black Pepper

120ml Tomato Ketchup

60ml Orange Juice

60ml Maple Syrup

1 Tablespoon Worcestershire Sauce

1 Tablespoon Apple Cider Vinegar

½ Teaspoon Paprika

3 Garlic Cloves Minced

Instructions

1. Onto a skewer thread 3 scallops and 3 shrimps alternately. Then brush with the vegetable before seasoning with the salt and pepper. Then place to one side for cooking later.

2. In to bowl put the ketchup, orange juice, maple syrup, Worcestershire sauce, apple cider vinegar, paprika and garlic and combine well together. This you will then be used for basting the scallops and shrimps as they cook on the barbecue. So set to onside until you start cooking.

3. Whilst you are doing the various tasks above you should be getting your barbecue started with the grill be set about 4 to 6 inches above the heat source so the food can cook on a medium to high heat.

4. As soon as your barbecue is ready lightly oil the grill and then place the shrimp and scallop kebabs on it. But just before you do brush the kebabs all over with the maple orange sauce and then baste them with it regularly. Each side of these kebabs should be allowed to cook for 2 to 3 minutes or until the flesh of the scallops and shrimps have turned opaque.

RECIPE 21 – GINGER SHRIMP WITH CHARRED TOMATO RELISH

Green tomatoes quite simply are ones that haven't ripened yet. Not only do they have slightly sour taste to them but also contain less sugar. By charring them you will find that they are a lot easier to peel because they have become softer.

Barbecue Cookbook

Ingredients

20 Extra Large Shrimps (Peeled, Deveined but Tails Left On)

2 Garlic Cloves Minced

1 ½ Tablespoons Grated Peeled Ginger

3 Tablespoons Vegetable Oil

4 Ripe Plum Tomatoes (Cut In Half Lengthwise)

2 Medium Green Tomatoes (Cut In Half Lengthwise)

Coarse Salt

Freshly Ground Black Pepper

2 Tablespoons Fresh Lime Juice

1 Tablespoon Freshly Minced Jalapeno Chilli (With Seeds)

1 Teaspoon Sugar

1 Tablespoon Freshly Chopped Cilantro

1 Tablespoon Freshly Chopped Basil

Instructions

1. In to a bowl mix together the garlic and ginger. Now take half of this and transfer to another bowl and add to these 2 tablespoons of the oil before then adding the shrimps and tossing them in the mixture to make sure that they are evenly coated in it. Now cover this bowl over and place in the refrigerator for 30 minutes to allow the shrimps to marinate. As for the rest of the ginger and garlic

mixture this should be covered and placed in the refrigerator as well.

2. Now heat up the barbecue and whilst this is happening into another bowl put the tomatoes and toss them in the last tablespoon of oil along with some salt and pepper to season. Now grill the tomatoes on the barbecue the cut sides facing upwards until the skins become charred and the flesh inside becomes tender.

The plum tomatoes will take around 4 to 6 minutes to cook and the green tomatoes will take about 8 to 10 minutes to cook. If the green tomatoes are especially hard they may need a little longer than 10 minutes.

Also be careful when cooking the tomatoes as both the juices from them and the oil in which they are coated may cause flare ups to occur.

3. Once the skins have become charred on the tomatoes and the flesh soft remove from heat and set to one side to allow them to cool down a little. As soon as they have cooled down enough peel away and discard the skins and seeds then finely chop them up and add to the garlic and ginger mixture from earlier. Also add to this mixture the lime juice, jalapeno chili, sugar cilantro and basil then well combined together pour into a serving dish and set to one side for later.

4. Remove shrimps from refrigerator and just before placing on to the barbecue thread one shrimp on to a skewer through both the top and tail and sprinkle with some salt and pepper. Place on the barbecue and cook for about 2 minutes on each side or until the flesh has turned opaque throughout.

Once cooked place the skewers on to a clean plate along with the bowl of tomato relish you made earlier.

Barbecue Cookbook

RECIPE 22 – SHRIMP & BROCCOLI PACKETS

If you want to serve your guests with a flavorsome but fuss free meal then this one should be considered.

Ingredients

225grams Medium Size Shrimps (Peeled and Deveined)

175grams Instant Rice

2 Teaspoons Seafood Seasoning

2 Garlic Cloves Minced

220grams Broccoli Florets

2 Tablespoons Butter (Cut Into Pieces)

8 Ice Cubes

120ml Water

Instructions

1. Preheat the barbecue and place the grill about 4 to 6 inches above the heat source so you can cook these parcels on a medium to high heat.

2. Whilst the barbecue is heating up place half the shrimps on a piece of aluminum foil with the nonstick (dull) side facing up towards the food. Then around this arrange half the rice and sprinkle it and the shrimps with some of the seafood seasoning before then topping off the shrimps with half the minced garlic.

Then place half the broccoli on top of the shrimp and sprinkle with garlic and butter. Do the same for the other parcel and then top each one off with 4 ice cubes.

3. Now bring the sides of the aluminum foil up and double fold over the top and at one end. At the end, which is still open, pour in half the water and then fold this end over so that the ingredients are now sealed inside. Make sure that you use a large enough piece of foil to allow room for heat and steam to circulate inside.

4. Once the parcels are ready place on the barbecue and let them cook for 9 to 13 minutes. It is important that you close the lid whilst the parcels are cooking to ensure that things cook evenly.

5. After removing from the grill snip open the parcels and stir the rice before you then serve as they are to your guests. It is also a good idea to squeeze some fresh lemon juice over the shrimps, rice and broccoli just before serving.

RECIPE 23 – TANGY SHRIMP & SCALLOPS

After cooking serve these kebabs with pasta, green salad and some garlic bread.

Ingredients

28 Large Shrimps (Peeled & Deveined)

28 Large Sea Scallops

113grams Butter or Margarine

7 Tablespoons Lemon Juice (Fresh Would Be Ideal)

Barbecue Cookbook

5 Tablespoons Worcestershire Sauce

1 Teaspoon Garlic Powder

1 Teaspoon Paprika

Instructions

1. In a large resealable bag place the scallops and shrimps.

2. Now into a bowl (that can be used safely in a microwave) place the butter or margarine, the lemon juice, Worcestershire sauce, garlic powder and paprika. Cook on 50% power for about 1 to 1 ½ minutes or until the butter/margarine is melted then stir to ensure that all these ingredients are blended together.

3. Once the sauce is made set aside about a third of it as this you will then use to baste the shrimps and scallops in whilst they are cooking. As for the rest of the sauce this must be poured over the scallops and shrimps in the bag. Now seal the bag and turn it over several times to ensure that every scallop and shrimp is coated in the sauce and place in the refrigerator for one hour. Whilst in the refrigerator make sure that you turn the back over occasionally.

3. Whilst the barbecue is heating up you can now prepare the kebabs. Take some wooden skewers that have been soaking in water and thread alternately on to them the scallops and shrimps.

4. Once all the kebabs are made place them on the preheated barbecue and cook them on a medium to hot heat for 6 minutes turning once during this time. Both before and during this cooking time baste them occasionally with the sauce you set to one side earlier. Then cook them for a further 8 to 10 minutes or longer until the shrimps have turned pink and the scallops opaque.

Recipe 24 – Barbecued Oysters Served With Hogwash

Looking for something special to serve at your next barbecue to your guests then why not give this recipe a go.

Ingredients

48 Oysters (Scrubbed)

Hogwash

120ml Natural Rice Vinegar

120ml Seasoned Rice Vinegar

2 Finely Chopped Shallots

3 Tablespoons Freshly Squeezed (Strained) Lime Juice

1 Small Jalapeno Chili (Seeded and Finely Chopped)

Fresh Roughly Chopped Cilantro

Instructions

1. Heat up the barbecue until it is very hot then place the unopened fresh oysters on to the lightly oiled grill and close the lid. After about 3 minutes check to see if the oysters are open.

2. If the oysters are open then detach the oysters from the top shell using an oyster knife. Then loosen the top shells and discard

these. Then you simply need to place a spoonful of the Hogwash sauce you have made over each one before serving them.

3. In order to make the Hogwash place the seasoned and natural rice vinegar into a bowl with the shallots, lime juice, jalapeno chili and cilantro and mix well together. You should make this before you actually begin cooking the oysters, as it needs to go into the refrigerator for at least an hour.

Recipe 25 – Scallops, Orange & Cucumber Kebabs

Yet another very simple recipe you may want to try but is one that really helps to enhance the amazing flavors of the scallops. It is important that you use the freshest scallops possible.

Ingredients

450grams Large Scallops

8 Very Thin Slices Peeled Fresh Ginger

2 Tablespoons Honey

120ml Fresh Orange Juice

½ Navel Orange Cut Into Wedges

½ Cucumber Cut In Half Lengthways Then Cut Into ½ Inch Slices

Coarse Salt

Freshly Ground Black Pepper

Samantha Michaels

Instructions

1. Start by getting the barbecue heated up. You will need to place the lightly oiled grill about 6 inches above the heat source as you want to cook these kebabs on a medium heat to ensure that nothing burns.

2. Whilst the barbecue is heating up in a small bowl mix together the honey and orange juice and set to one side for later.

3. Next take four skewers (wooden ones will do but you can use metal ones if you want). On to these thread an orange wedge followed by a slice of ginger, cucumber and scallop until each skewer is full. Also make sure that you end with another wedge of orange on the kebabs.

4. Now season each kebab with salt and pepper before then brushing with the orange and honey sauce made earlier. Place each kebab on to the grill of the barbecue and cook for between 4 and 6 minutes or until the scallop flesh has turned opaque. Make sure that you turn the kebabs frequently and baste regularly with the sauce.

Once the kebabs are cooked serve with some rice or a crisp green salad.

RECIPE 26 – PRAWNS WITH PISTOU

If you wish rather than using prawns you can use large shrimps instead.

Ingredients

12 Prawns (Shelled and Deveined But With Heads Left On)

27.5grams Whole Raw Almonds

128grams Loose Packed Fresh Flat Leaf Parsley

12 Anchovy Fillets (Rinsed)

2 Garlic Cloves (Peeled)

60ml Extra Virgin Olive Oil

2 Tablespoons Extra Virgin Olive Oil

Zest of 1 Lemon

Coarse Salt

Freshly Ground Black Pepper

Instructions

1. Take the whole raw almonds and place in the oven on a baking tray for 10 minutes at 350 degrees Fahrenheit. Stir the almonds occasionally and remove from oven when golden brown and fragrant. Then allow to cool down completely before coarsely chopping them.

2. Now take the coarsely chopped almonds and place them in food processor with the basil, parsley, anchovies and garlic and process until all have been combined together. Then to this paste add the oil very slowly in a steady stream and continue processing until a smooth paste is formed.

Now transfer this mixture to a large bowl and mix in the lemon zest, salt and pepper. Put around a ¼ of this mixture to one side, as this is what your guests will then dip the shrimps in after they are cooked.

3. Whilst you are preparing the Pistou you should be allowing the barbecue to heat up ready for cooking. Place the grill about 5 inches above the heat source, as you will want to cook the shrimps on a medium to high heat.

4. As soon as the barbecue is ready toss the shrimps in the rest of the Pistou and place them on the barbecue and cook for about 2 ½ minutes on each side. Plus before placing on the barbecue season with some salt and pepper. You should only turn the shrimps over once during the cooking time and to make sure that they are cooked through the flesh should be firm and they should have turned pink.

5. As soon as the shrimps are cooked place onto a clean plate with some lemon wedges and the bowl of Pistou you put to one side earlier. Your guests can then dip the shrimps into this.

RECIPE 27 – BLACK & WHITE PEPPER SHRIMPS

If you can use sustainable peppercorns for this particular recipe. You are going to find that this is a recipe that will prove a favorite with everyone.

Ingredients

450grams Jumbo Shrimps (Heads Still On But Peeled & Deveined)

1 Tablespoon Black Peppercorns

2 Teaspoons White Peppercorns

1 ½ Tablespoons Maldon Sea Salt

3 Tablespoons Safflower Oil

8 Sprigs Fresh Cilantro For Garnish

Instructions

1. In a shallow dish place 8 wooden skewers measuring 10 inches in cold water for at least 10 minutes.

2. Now start the barbecue up putting the grill about 6 inches above the heat source so that the shrimps can cook on a medium to high heat.

3. Whilst the barbecue is heating up thread the shrimps on to the skewers starting with at the tail and threading through the body until it comes out of the head. Now put each one of these on to a baking tray for now.

4. In a mortar place the peppercorns and coarsely grind them together with a pestle. Then transfer these to a small bowl and mix into them the sea salt.

5. Just before you place the shrimps on the barbecue drizzle them with the oil (both sides) and then sprinkle with the peppercorn and salt mixture.

6. Now place the shrimps on the lightly oiled barbecue grill and cook until the prawns become a light pink color and slightly charred. This should take around 2 minutes to occur then turn the shrimps over and cook for about the same amount of time again.

7. To serve place the shrimps on a place and sprinkle with the sprigs of cilantro and a dipping sauce in a bowl.

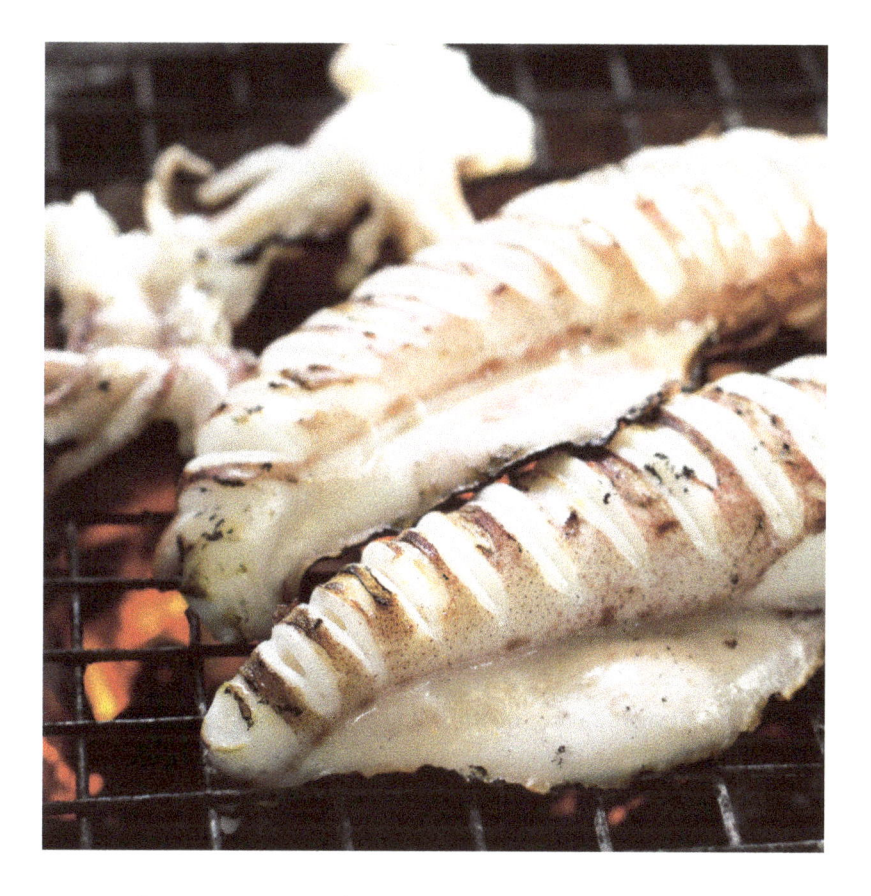

RECIPE 28 – GRILLED CALAMARI

To avoid your calamari from becoming too chewy you need to either cook it really fast or really slow. When cooked serve it in a large bowl or as individual servings to your guests.

Barbecue Cookbook

Ingredients

450grams Fresh Calamari (Cleaned, Rinsed & Well Dried)

60ml Extra Virgin Olive Oil

1 ½ Tablespoons Fresh Lemon Juice (About 1 Small Lemon)

1 Garlic Clove Thinly Sliced

2 Sprigs of Fresh Oregano or ½ Teaspoon Dried Oregano

½ Teaspoon Coarse Salt

Freshly Ground Black Pepper

Instructions

1. In a bowl place the olive oil; lemon juice and salt then stir until they combined together. Then Into this mix the garlic and the whole sprigs or dried oregano.

2. Whilst you are making up this sauce you should be getting the barbecue heated up and place the grill down as low as possible in order to cook the calamari quick on a very high heat.

3. When the barbecue has heated up place the squid on the oiled grill and char each side of it for 1 minute. Now remove from the barbecue and slice all parts of the calamari including the tendrils cross wise into ¼ inch rings. Then add the calamari to the lemon sauce made earlier and then place on a serving plate. Just before you serve this dish to your guests make sure that you sprinkle over some freshly ground black pepper.

RECIPE JOURNAL

RECIPE #1

RECIPE: _____

Ingredients:

-
-
-
-
-
-
-
-

-
-
-
-
-
-
-
-

Directions:

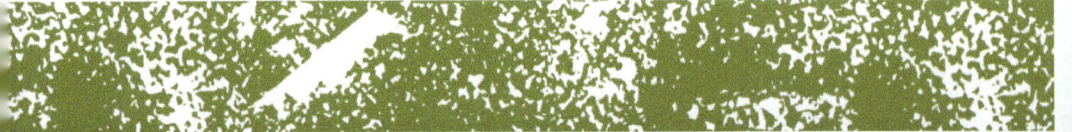

Preparation Time: **Servings:**

RECIPE #2

RECIPE: _____

Ingredients:

- _____
- _____
- _____
- _____
- _____
- _____
- _____
- _____

- _____
- _____
- _____
- _____
- _____
- _____
- _____
- _____

Directions:

_____
_____
_____
_____
_____
_____
_____
_____
_____
_____
_____
_____
_____
_____

Preparation Time: **Servings:**

RECIPE #3

RECIPE: _____

Ingredients:

-
-
-
-
-
-
-
-

-
-
-
-
-
-
-
-

Directions:

Preparation Time: **Servings:**

RECIPE #4

RECIPE: _____

Ingredients:

- .... - ....
- .... - ....
- .... - ....
- .... - ....
- .... - ....
- .... - ....
- .... - ....
- ....

Directions:

....
....
....
....
....
....
....
....
....
....
....
....

Preparation Time: **Servings:**

RECIPE #5

RECIPE: _____

Ingredients:

- ....
- ....
- ....
- ....
- ....
- ....
- ....
- ....

- ....
- ....
- ....
- ....
- ....
- ....
- ....
- ....

Directions:

....
....
....
....
....
....
....
....
....
....
....
....

Preparation Time: **Servings:**

RECIPE #6

RECIPE: _____

Ingredients:

-
-
-
-
-
-
-
-

-
-
-
-
-
-
-
-

Directions:

Preparation Time: **Servings:**

RECIPE #7

RECIPE: _____

Ingredients:

- ....
- ....
- ....
- ....
- ....
- ....
- ....
- ....

- ....
- ....
- ....
- ....
- ....
- ....
- ....
- ....

Directions:

....

....

....

....

....

....

....

....

....

....

....

....

....

Preparation Time: **Servings:**

RECIPE #8

RECIPE: _____

Ingredients:

- ....
- ....
- ....
- ....
- ....
- ....
- ....
- ....

- ....
- ....
- ....
- ....
- ....
- ....
- ....
- ....

Directions:

....
....
....
....
....
....
....
....
....
....
....
....
....
....

Preparation Time: **Servings:**

RECIPE #9

RECIPE: _____

Ingredients:

- ....
- ....
- ....
- ....
- ....
- ....
- ....
- ....

- ....
- ....
- ....
- ....
- ....
- ....
- ....
- ....

Directions:

Preparation Time: **Servings:**

RECIPE #10

RECIPE: _____

Ingredients:

-
-
-
-
-
-
-

-
-
-
-
-
-
-

Directions:

Preparation Time: **Servings:**

RECIPE #11

RECIPE: _____

Ingredients:

- ....
- ....
- ....
- ....
- ....
- ....
- ....
- ....

- ....
- ....
- ....
- ....
- ....
- ....
- ....

Directions:

....
....
....
....
....
....
....
....
....
....
....
....
....

Preparation Time: **Servings:**

RECIPE #12

RECIPE: _____

Ingredients:

- ....
- ....
- ....
- ....
- ....
- ....
- ....
- ....

- ....
- ....
- ....
- ....
- ....
- ....
- ....
- ....

Directions:

....
....
....
....
....
....
....
....
....
....
....
....
....
....

Preparation Time: **Servings:**

# RECIPE #13

RECIPE: _____

Ingredients:

- ....
- ....
- ....
- ....
- ....
- ....
- ....
- ....

- ....
- ....
- ....
- ....
- ....
- ....
- ....
- ....

Directions:

....
....
....
....
....
....
....
....
....
....
....
....
....
....

Preparation Time: **Servings:**

RECIPE #14

RECIPE: _____

Ingredients:

- ....
- ....
- ....
- ....
- ....
- ....
- ....
- ....

- ....
- ....
- ....
- ....
- ....
- ....
- ....
- ....

Directions:

....
....
....
....
....
....
....
....
....
....
....
....
....
....

Preparation Time: **Servings:**

RECIPE #15

RECIPE: _____

Ingredients:

-
-
-
-
-
-
-
-

-
-
-
-
-
-
-
-

Directions:

Preparation Time: **Servings:**

RECIPE #16

RECIPE: _____

Ingredients:

- ....
- ....
- ....
- ....
- ....
- ....
- ....
- ....

- ....
- ....
- ....
- ....
- ....
- ....
- ....
- ....

Directions:

....
....
....
....
....
....
....
....
....
....
....
....
....
....

Preparation Time: **Servings:**

RECIPE #17

RECIPE: _____

Ingredients:

- ....
- ....
- ....
- ....
- ....
- ....
- ....
- ....

- ....
- ....
- ....
- ....
- ....
- ....
- ....
- ....

Directions:

....
....
....
....
....
....
....
....
....
....
....
....
....
....
....

Preparation Time: **Servings:**

RECIPE #18

RECIPE: _____

Ingredients:

-
-
-
-
-
-
-

-
-
-
-
-
-
-

Directions:

Preparation Time: **Servings:**

RECIPE #19

RECIPE: _____

Ingredients:

- ....
- ....
- ....
- ....
- ....
- ....
- ....
- ....

- ....
- ....
- ....
- ....
- ....
- ....
- ....

Directions:

....
....
....
....
....
....
....
....
....
....
....
....
....

Preparation Time: **Servings:**

RECIPE #20

RECIPE: _____

Ingredients:

- ....
- ....
- ....
- ....
- ....
- ....
- ....
- ....

- ....
- ....
- ....
- ....
- ....
- ....
- ....

Directions:

....
....
....
....
....
....
....
....
....
....
....
....
....

Preparation Time: **Servings:**

About The Author

Samantha Michaels has spent years helping people overcome health challenges, lose weight and reach ideal health goals while enjoying good and healthy food. She is an author of numerous health books and provide amazing yet very healthy recipes everyone can enjoy.

She loves food and spends most of her time helping people address diet challenges by teaching them to cook the right meals. Her diet programs have helped a lot of people lose weight in a smart, practical way and she lives what she preaches that you do not have to get hungry while on a diet.